# DEJA REVIEW™

## Internal Medicine

# NOTICE

# DEJA REVIEW™
## Internal Medicine

**Second Edition**

## Sarvenaz S. Saadat Mobasser, MD

School of Medicine
University of California, Irvine
Irvine, California
Residency in Family Medicine
Kaiser Permanente
Woodland Hills Medical Center
Woodland Hills, California

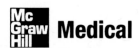 **Medical**

New York   Chicago   San Francisco   Lisbon   London   Madrid   Mexico City
Milan   New Delhi   San Juan   Seoul   Singapore   Sydney   Toronto

## Déjà Review™: Internal Medicine, Second Edition

2 3 4 5 6 7 8 9 10   IBT/IBT   1 9 8 7 6 5 4 3 2

ISBN 978-0-07-171517-1
MHID 0-07-171517-7

This book was set in Palatino by Glyph International.

The editors were Kirsten Funk and Cindy Yoo.

The production supervisor was Catherine H. Saggese.

Project management was provided by Harleen Chopra, Glyph International

IBT Global was printer and binder.

This book is printed on acid-free paper.

Library of Congress Cataloging-in-Publication Data

Mobasser, Sarvenaz S. Saadat, author.
  Deja review. Internal medicine / Sarvenaz S. Saadat Mobasser, MD, School of Medicine, University of California, Irvine, Irvine, California, Completed Residency in Family Medicine, Kaiser Permanente, Woodland Hills Medical Center, Woodland Hills, California.—Second Edition.
        p. ; cm.—(Deja review)
     Internal medicine
     Includes index.
     ISBN-13: 978-0-07-171517-1 (pbk. : alk. paper)
     ISBN-10: 0-07-171517-7 (pbk. : alk. paper)   1. Internal medicine—Examinations, questions, etc.   I. Title. II. Title: Internal medicine.   III. Series: Deja review.
     [DNLM: 1. Internal Medicine—Examination Questions.   WB 18.2]
     RC58.S33   2011
     616.0076—dc22

                                                                        2010050479

McGraw-Hill books are available at special quantity discounts to use as premiums and sales promotions, or for use in corporate training programs. To contact a representative please e-mail us at bulksales@mcgraw-hill.com.

*To my beautiful daughters Chaya and Charlotte:*
*You are the inspiration for everything I do.*
*You put the twinkle in my eyes.*
*Always reach for the moon and the stars!*
*With all my love,*
*Mommy*

# Contents

# Reviewers

**Edward R. Gould**
Fourth Year Medical Student
SUNY Upstate Medical University
Class of 2009

**Michael Sidholm, MD**
PGY-1 Internal Medicine
Ross University
School of Medicine
Class of 2008

**Robert Nastasi, MS**
PGY-1
SUNY Upstate Medical University
Class of 2008

**Vivek Punjabi, MD**
PGY-1
UMDNJ
Class of 2008

# Acknowledgments

The author would like to acknowledge the following individuals for their work on the first edition:

*Image Contributors:*
Noah Craft, MD, PhD, DTM&H
William Herring, MD, FACR
Henry J. Feldman, MD

*Reviewers:*
Daniel Behroozan, MD
Paul Bellamy, MD
Jia-ling Chou, MD
Afshin Khatibi, MD
Rashmi Nadig
Pamela Nagami, MD
Braden Nago, MD
Frederick Ziel, MD

# Preface

The principles learned in *internal medicine* are the fundamental core principles applied in clinical medicine as well as the largest proportion of questions posed on the USMLE Step 2CK exam. In order to do well both on the wards and on the Step 2CK exam, you must have a solid foundation in these principles. This guide has been written as a high-yield resource to endorse the rapid recall of the essential facts in a well-organized and efficient manner.

## ORGANIZATION

All concepts are presented in a question and answer format that covers the key facts on hundreds of commonly tested internal medicine topics that may appear on the USMLE Step 2CK exam. The material is divided into chapters organized by internal medicine subcategories, along with vignettes at the end of each chapter that incorporate the material with their clinical presentation and relevance.

This question and answer format has several advantages:

- It provides a rapid, straightforward way for you to assess your strengths and weaknesses.
- It allows you to efficiently review and commit to memory a large body of information.
- The clinical vignettes incorporated expose you to the prototypical presentation of diseases classically tested on USMLE Step 2CK.
- It serves as a quick, last-minute review of high-yield facts.
- Compact, condensed design of the book is conducive to studying on the go.

## HOW TO USE THIS BOOK

This text is intended to be used not only to study for the USMLE Step 2CK exam but is also an essential tool while on the internal medicine and medicine subspecialty rotations, and during medical school. Remember, this text is not intended to replace comprehensive textbooks, course packets, or lectures. It is simply intended to serve as a supplement to your studies during your internal medicine clinical rotation and throughout your preparation for Step 2CK. We encourage you to begin using this book early in your third year to reinforce topics you encounter while on the wards. Also, it is recommended that you cover up the answers (rather than just reading both the questions and the answers) and quiz yourself or even your classmates. Carry the book in

| | |
|---|---|
| Protein, total | 6.7-8.2 g/dL |
| PSA, age age 0-39 | 0-1.4 ng/mL |
| PSA, age age 40+ | 0-2.8 ng/mL |
| Reticulocyte count | 0.5%-1.5% |
| SGOT | 10-42 U/L |
| SGPT | <60 U/L |
| Sodium | 135-145 mEq/L |
| T3 uptake | 25%-38% |
| T4 total | 0.7-2.1 ng/dL |
| Transferrin | 212-360 mg/dL |
| TSH | 0.5-5.0 µIU/mL |
| Uric acid | 2.6-7.2 mg/dL |
| WBC | 4500-10,500 |

## Writing Notes

**Daily progress note**: This should be in SOAP format.

**Subjective:** In this area you should report any overnight events, how the patient is feeling today, any complaints or problems the patient may be experiencing, and pertinent positives and negatives.

**Objective:** Any physical findings are reported in this section.

Vitals: temperature, max temperature, blood pressure, pulse, respiratory rate, oxygen saturation

Glucose (if patient is diabetic): Ins and Outs (Ins = IV fluids + po intake + any parenteral intake or blood products over 24 hours and Outs = urine output + stool + other [NG tube, chest tube, drains, emesis])

Physical examination:
    General: Patient's general appearance
    HEENT (head, eyes, ears, nose, throat)
    Cardiovascular
    Pulmonary
    Abdomen
    Extremities
    Neurologic

Labs: Laboratory tests are reported here.

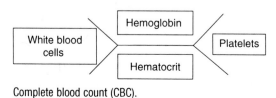

Complete blood count (CBC).

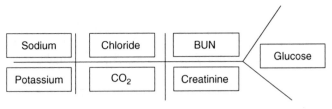

Chemistry 7.

**Meds**: Some people include a list of all the medication the patient is currently using. **Assessment** and **plan**: Write a summary of the patient, their problem(s) and possible differentials. Then write the plan for each problem.

X

*Sign your note*

### Example

S: Patient has no complaints today. She is no longer short of breath and was able to ambulate yesterday.

O: T: 36.8°C, Tmax 37°C, P: 70-85, BP: 128-148/68-80, RR: 20, $O_2$ sat: 95-100%, I/O: 1500/2000

GEN: NAD (no apparent distress)

HEENT: PERRLA (pupils are equally round and reactive to light accommodation), EOMI (extraocular muscles are intact), NCAT (normocephalic atraumatic)

CV: RRR no M/R/G (regular rate and rhythm with no murmurs, rubs, or gallops)

Pulm: CTA B (clear to auscultation bilaterally); no R/R/W (no rhonchi, rales, or wheezes)

Abd: S (soft)/NT (nontender)/ND (nondistended)/NABS (normal abdominal bowel sounds)

Ext: no C (clubbing)/C (cyanosis)/E (edema); no calf tenderness

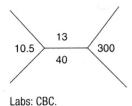

Labs: CBC.

Meds: Aspirin 81 mg daily
     Albuterol nebs q4h

A/P: 35 y/o female with asthma exacerbation now improved and at baseline

1. Asthma: Patient improved with steroids and albuterol/atrovent treatments. Patient will be sent home with a medrol pack and albuterol inhaler. Patient will also be sent home with a steroid inhaler.
2. Disposition: Patient will be discharged home today with follow-up in 1 week.

*Greta Student, MS III*

## History and Physical Examination

**Chief complaint (CC):** Main problem that the patient is here for (eg, shortness of breath)

**History of present illness (HPI):** Include a chronologic history of the patient's problems and prior treatments for this problem as well as any other history that is pertinent. Describe symptoms in terms of onset, duration, quality of discomfort, setting, instigating and relieving factors.

**Past medical history (PMH):** Include the patient's medical history and be sure to ask about heart disease, hypertension, diabetes, cancer, and any other pertinent history. The patient's medication list can often serve as a clue since patients will sometimes forget to mention medical problems that they have.

**Surgical history (SH):** Include all operations a patient has as well as when and why. **Medication:** List all the patient's medications as well as doses and frequency with which they are taken. Also ask the patient about any possible over-the-counter medications and alternative meds.

**Allergies:** Name all drugs the patient is allergic to and what happened when they took the drug.

NKDA means "no known drug allergies"

**Family history (FH):** This should include the health, medical problems of the patient's family including parents, grandparents, siblings, and often, aunts, uncles, and cousins. Be sure to ask about heart disease, diabetes, hypertension, hyperlipidemia, and cancer.

**Social history (SH):** This section includes the patient's marital status, occupation, exercise history, sexual history, diet, and tobacco use, drug use, and alcohol use.

**Review of systems (ROS):** Report all the pertinent positive and negative signs and symptoms that the patient reports (eg, the patient denies any nausea, vomiting, diarrhea, chest pain, cough, travel history . . . )

**Physical examination:** Include all pertinent organs and systems:

Vital signs: Tmax, BP, HR, RR, $O_2$ sat, Ins/Outs
General:
HEENT:
Neck:

Cardiovascular:
Pulmonary:
Abdominal:
Genitourinary:
Back:
Extremities:
Neurologic:

**Labs and studies:** Include all labs and studies that you have results for.
Assesment and plan: Write a summary of the patient's problems and differential diagnoses as well as a plan for each problem.
X
*Sign your name at the bottom*

## Procedure Note

Whenever a procedure is done, a procedure note must be written in the chart. Always remember to get consent from the patient before a procedure is done. Below is an example.

**Procedure Note:**

Procedure: Biopsy of left lower abdominal macule.

Indications: Rule out melanoma.

Consent: The risks, benefits, and possible side effects of the procedure including but not exclusive of pain, bleeding, infection, and scar were explained to the patient who understands and wishes to have the procedure done.

Preparation: The area was prepped and draped in a sterile fashion.

Anesthesia: The area was anesthetized with 10 cc of 2% lidocaine solution using a 30-gauge needle.

Procedure: A wide excision (1 cm on each side) of the macule was done using a number-15 blade. There was minimal bleeding. The site of the excision was closed using 4-0 nylon sutures and the specimen was sent to pathology for examination.

Complications: The patient tolerated the procedure with no complications.

*Greta Student, MS III*

## How to Write a Prescription

Patient name: _____ Medical record number_____
Address:_____ Phone #:_____DOB:_____

Rx: *Drug name, drug dose*
    Dispense # : Write number here
    Sig: Write instructions here
    Refill:

X *Sign your name here*                              Date:_____

Example

Patient name: Ima N. Payne_____ Medical record number: 12345678
Address: 1111 Oak Street ; LA, CA Phone #: 222-2222   DOB:1/1/69_____
Rx: Famotidine 20 mg tablets
    Dispense # : Sixty
    Sig: Take two tablets by mouth twice daily
    Refill: 1
X *Dr. Health*                                       Date: 10/20/09

## How to Admit a Patient

Admission Orders

Admit to:
  Floor:
  Service:
  Medical student name:
  Resident name:
  Attending name:
Diagnosis:
  Primary diagnosis:
  Other diagnoses:
Condition:
  Good, stable, fair, guarded, critical
Vitals:
  Per routine (usually q2h in ICU and q4h on the floor)
  q shift
  q __ h

Activity:
  Ad lib
  Bed rest
  To chair
  Ambulate bid
  Bathroom privileges
  Fall risk
Nursing:
  Neuro check q__h
  Weigh daily
  Pulse oximetry
  Wound care
  CALL MD for systolic blood pressure (SBP) >165 or <110; diastolic BP >100 or <60; Pulse >100, T >38.5°C
  Etc
Diet:
  Regular
  Diabetic
  Low sodium
  Low fat
  Clear liquid
  Soft
  npo (nothing by mouth)
Ins and Outs: strict, per routine
  IV fluids: eg, D51/2NS @ 100 cc/h
  Drains: Foley, NG tube to suction, chest tube to suction
Medication:
  Medication name, dose, route, frequency
  Home medication should be written out
  Antibiotics
  Etc
Special: These are things you will usually need to think about.
  DVT prophylaxis
  Pain medications
  Antiemetics
  Antipyretics
Allergies:
  NKDA (no known drug allergies)
  Penicillin
  Sulfa
  Etc
Labs/studies:
  CBC, electrolytes, BUN, Cr, ECG, radiology studies; other labs

**Example**

> Admit to 2 North, Internal Medicine, Medical Student: Stew Dent;
> Resident:
> Dr. Smith; Attending: Dr. Bay
> Diagnosis: Pneumonia
> Condition: Fair
> Vitals: Per routine
> Activity: Bathroom privileges
> Nursing: Pulse oximetry; call MD for systolic blood pressure (SBP) > 165 or < 110;
> diastolic BP > 100 or < 60; Pulse > 100, Temp > 38.5; Pulse ox < 90%
> Diet: Regular
> Ins and outs: Strict
>      IV fluids: D5NS@120 cc/h
> Meds: Ceftriaxone 2 g IV q24 hours
>      Azithromycin 500 mg IV q24 hours
>      Tylenol 650 mg po q6 hours prn mild pain or Temp > 38.5
> Special: Sequential compression stockings
> Allergies: NKDA
> Labs/studies: PA and lateral CXR; sputum culture/ Gram stain; CBC; electrolytes;
> BUN; Cr

## Abbreviations You Should Know

| AAA | abdominal aortic aneurysm |
|---|---|
| AAS | acute abdominal series |
| abd | abdomen |
| Abx | antibiotics |
| ac | before meals |
| ACLS | advanced cardiac life support |
| ACTH | adrenocorticotropic hormone |
| ADA | American Diabetes Association |
| ADH | antidiuretic hormone |
| ADL | activities of daily living |
| AFB | acid fast bacillus |
| AFP | alpha feto protein |
| AI | aortic insufficiency |
| AKA | above knee amputation |
| alk phos | alkaline phosphatase |
| ALL | acute lymphocytic leukemia |
| ALS | amytrophic lateral sclerosis |
| AMA | against medical advice |
| AMI | acute myocardial infarction |

| | |
|---|---|
| AML | acute myelogenous leukemia |
| ANA | antinuclear antibody |
| ant | anterior |
| AP | anteroposterior |
| APTT | activated partial thromboplastin time |
| AR | aortic regurgitation |
| ARDS | acute respiratory distress syndrome |
| ARF | acute renal failure |
| AS | aortic stenosis |
| ASA | aspirin |
| ASD | atrial septal defect |
| ASO | antistreptolysin O |
| ATN | acute tubular necrosis |
| AV | arteriovenous |
| AVN | atrioventricular node |
| B | bilateral |
| BBB | bundle branch block |
| BE | barium enema |
| BIB | brought in by |
| bid | two times per day |
| BKA | below knee amputation |
| BM | bowel movement; bone marrow |
| BPH | benign prostatic hypertrophy |
| BRBPR | bright red blood per rectum |
| BRP | bathroom privileges |
| BS | blood sugar; breath sounds |
| BUN | blood urea nitrogen |
| Bx | biopsy |
| c | with |
| Ca | calcium |
| CA | cancer, carcinoma |
| CABG | coronary artery bypass graft |
| CAD | coronary artery disease |
| cath | catheter |
| CBC | complete blood count |
| CBG | capillary blood gas |
| CC | chief complaint |
| CEA | carcinoembryonic antigen |
| CF | cystic fibrosis |
| CHF | congestive heart failure |
| CK-MB | creatinine kinase-myocardial band |
| CLL | chronic lymphocytic leukemia |
| CML | chronic myelogenous leukemia |
| CMV | cytomegalovirus |
| CN | cranial nerves |

| | |
|---|---|
| CNS | central nervous system |
| CO | cardiac output |
| c/o | complains of |
| COPD | chronic obstructive pulmonary disease |
| CP | chest pain |
| CPAP | continuous positive airway pressure |
| CPK | creatinine phosphokinase |
| CPR | cardiopulmonary resuscitation |
| CRF | chronic renal failure |
| C and S | culture and sensitivity |
| CSF | cerebrospinal fluid |
| CT | computerized tomography |
| CTAB | clear to auscultation bilaterally |
| CV | cardiovascular |
| CVA | cerebrovascular accident |
| CVAT | costovertebral angle tenderness |
| CVP | central venous pressure |
| CXR | chest x-ray |
| D51/2NS | 5% dextrose in half normal saline |
| D5W | 5% dextrose in water |
| DA | dopamine |
| D/C | discharge, discontinue |
| Ddx | differential diagnosis |
| DI | diabetes insipidus |
| DIC | disseminated intravascular coagulation |
| DIP | distal interphalangeal joint |
| DJD | degenerative joint disease |
| DKA | diabetic ketoacidosis |
| DM | diabetes mellitus |
| DNR | do not resuscitate |
| DOA | dead on arrival |
| DOE | dyspnea on exertion |
| DT | delirium tremens |
| DTR | deep tendon reflexes |
| DVT | deep vein thrombosis |
| Dx | diagnosis |
| EBL | estimated blood loss |
| ECT | electroconvulsive therapy |
| EEG | electroencephalogram |
| EGD | esophagogastroduodenoscopy |
| EKG | electrocardiogram |
| EMG | electromyelogram |
| ENT | ears, nose, and throat |
| EOMI | extraocular muscles intact |
| ERCP | endoscopic retrograde cholangiopancreatography |

| | |
|---|---|
| ESR | erythrocyte sedimentation rate |
| ETOH | alcohol, ethanol |
| ETT | endotracheal tube |
| FB | foreign body |
| FBS | fasting blood sugar |
| f/c | fever and chills |
| $FEV_1$ | forced expiratory volume in 1 second |
| FFP | fresh frozen plasma |
| FH | family history |
| FRC | functional residual capacity |
| FTA-ABS | fluorescent treponemal antibody absorption (syphilis) |
| FTT | failure to thrive |
| f/u | follow-up |
| FUO | fever of unknown origin |
| FVC | forced vital capacity |
| fx | fracture |
| GC | gonococcus, gonorrhea |
| GERD | gastroesophageal reflux disease |
| GI | gastrointestinal |
| GU | genitourinary |
| HA | headache |
| HBsAg | hepatitis B surface antigen |
| HBV | hepatitis B virus |
| Hct | hematocrit |
| HDL | high-density lipoprotein |
| HEENT | head, eyes, ears, nose, throat |
| Hgb | hemoglobin |
| HIV | human immunodeficiency virus |
| HLA | histocompatablility locus antigen |
| h/o | history of |
| HO | house officer |
| HOB | head of bed |
| HPI | history of present illness |
| HSM | hepatosplenomegaly |
| HTN | hypertension |
| Hx | history |
| ICU | intensive care unit |
| I&D | incision and drainage |
| IDDM | insulin-dependent diabetes mellitus |
| Ig | immunoglobulin |
| IM | intramuscular |
| INH | isoniazid |
| I&O | intake and output |
| ITP | idopathic thrombocytopenic purpura |
| IVF | intravenous fluids |

| | |
|---|---|
| IVP | intravenous pyelogram |
| JVD | jugular venous distention |
| KUB | kidney ureter, bladder x-ray |
| LAD | left axis deviation (lymphadenopathy) |
| LAE | left atrial enlargement |
| LAP | left atrial pressure |
| LCM | left costal margin |
| LDH | lactate dehydrogenase |
| LLE | left lower extremity |
| LLL | left lower lobe |
| LLQ | left lower quadrant |
| LMN | lower motor neuron |
| LOC | loss of consciousness |
| LP | lumbar puncture |
| LR | lactated ringers |
| LUE | left upper extremity |
| LUL | left upper lobe |
| LUQ | left upper quadrant |
| LVH | left ventricular hypertrophy |
| m | murmur |
| MAO | monoamine oxidase inhibitor |
| MAP | mean arterial pressure |
| MCH | mean cell hemoglobin |
| MCHC | mean cell hemoglobin concentration |
| MCP | metacarpophalangeal joint |
| MCV | mean corpuscular volume |
| MEN | multiple endocrine neoplasia |
| MI | myocardial infarction |
| MRSA | methicillin-resistant *Staphylococcus aureus* |
| MS | mitral stenosis, multiple sclerosis |
| MVA | motor vehicle accident |
| MVI | multivitamin |
| NAD | no apparent distress |
| ND | nondistended |
| NG | nasogastric tube |
| NIDDM | non-insulin-dependant diabetes mellitus |
| NKDA | no known drug allergies |
| npo | nothing by mouth |
| NS | normal saline |
| NSAID | nonsteroidal anti-inflammatory drug |
| NSR | normal sinus rhythm |
| NT | nontender |
| N/V | nausea and vomiting |
| OB | occult blood |
| OOB | out of bed |

| | |
|---|---|
| OR | operating room |
| PAC | premature atrial contraction |
| PAT | paroxysmal atrial tachycardia |
| PCWP | pulmonary capillary wedge pressure |
| PDA | patent ductus arteriosus |
| PE | pulmonary embolism |
| PEEP | positive end-expiratory pressure |
| PERRLA | pupils equally round and reactive to light |
| PFT | pulmonary function test |
| PMD | primary medical doctor |
| PMH | past medical history |
| PMI | point of maximal impulse |
| PMN | polymorphonuclear cell |
| PM&R | physical medicine and rehabilitation |
| PND | paroxysmal nocturnal dyspnea |
| po | by mouth |
| POD | post operative day |
| PR | per rectum |
| PRBC | packed red blood cells |
| PT | physical therapy, prothrombin time |
| pt | patient |
| PTCA | percutaneous transluminal coronary angioplasty |
| PTH | parathyroid hormone |
| PTT | partial thromboplastin time |
| PUD | peptic ulcer disease |
| PVC | premature ventricular contraction |
| PVD | peripheral vascular disease |
| qAC | before each meal |
| qd | daily |
| qid | four times per day |
| qod | every other day |
| q4h | every 4 hours |
| RA | rheumatoid arthritis |
| RAD | right axis deviation |
| RAE | right atrial enlargement |
| RBC | red blood cells |
| RDW | red cell distribution width |
| RHD | rheumatic heart disease |
| RLE | right lower extremity |
| RLL | right lower lobe |
| RLQ | right lower quadrant |
| RML | right middle lobe |
| r/o | rule out |
| ROM | range of motion |
| ROS | review of systems |

| RR | respiratory rate |
| RRR | regular rate and rhythm |
| RT | respiratory therapy |
| RTA | renal tubular acidosis |
| RTC | return to clinic |
| RUE | right upper extremity |
| RUL | right upper lobe |
| RUQ | right upper quadrant |
| RVH | right ventricular hypertrophy |
| s | without |
| SBE | subacute bacterial endocarditis |
| SBO | small bowel obstruction |
| SBP | subacute bacterial peritonitis |
| SEM | systolic ejection murmur |
| SGOT | serum glutamic-oxaloacetic transaminase |
| SGPT | serum glutamic-pyruvic transaminase |
| SIADH | syndrome of inappropriate antidiuretic hormone |
| SL | sublingual |
| SLE | systemic lupus erythematosus |
| SOB | shortness of breath |
| s/p | status post |
| stat | immediate |
| subQ | subcutaneous |
| Sx | symptoms |
| T | temperature |
| tab | tablets |
| TB | tuberculosis |
| TIA | transient ischemic attack |
| TIBC | total iron-binding capacity |
| tid | three times per day |
| TKO | to keep open |
| TLC | total lung capacity |
| TPN | total parenteral nutrition |
| TSH | thyroid-stimulating hormone |
| TTP | thrombotic thrombocytopenic purpura |
| TURP | transurethral resection of the prostate |
| TV | total volume |
| Tx | Treatment |
| UA | Urinalysis |
| UGI | upper gastrointestinal |
| UMN | upper motor neuron |
| URI | upper respiratory infection |
| US | Ultrasound |
| UTI | urinary tract infection |
| VC | vital capacity |

VCUG voiding cystourethrogram
VDRL venereal disease research laboratory (syphilis test)
V/Q ventilation perfusion scan
VSS vital signs stable
WBC white blood cells
WNL within normal limits
y/o years old

## Common Formulas

Maintenance fluids per hour: 4:2:1 rule:

4 mL/kg up to 10 kg + 2 mL/kg from 11 to 30 kg + 1 mL/kg >30 kg
**Example:** A person weighing 100 kg should get

$(4 \times 10) + (2 \times 20) + (1 \times 70) = 40 + 40 + 70 = 150$ cc/h

Maintenance fluids over 24 hours: 100:50:20 rule

100 mL/kg up to 10 kg + 50 mL/kg from 11 to 30 kg + 20 mL/kg >30 kg

Anion gap: $Na - (Cl + HCO_3)$

Osmolality: $2Na + glucose/18 + BUN/2.8$

Fractional Na excretion $(FE_{Na})$ : $\dfrac{\text{urine Na} \times \text{serum creatinine}}{\text{serum Na} \times \text{urine creatinine}}$

Creatinine clearance, also known as glomerular filtration rate (GFR):

$$\frac{\text{urine creatinine} \times \text{urine volume in mL}}{\text{serum creatinine} \times \text{time in minutes}}$$

Estimated creatinine clearance : $\dfrac{(140 - \text{age}) \times (\text{weight in kg}) \,(\text{for females} \times 0.85)}{\text{serum creatinine} \times 72}$

Corrected Na: $Na + [(\text{glucose} - 100) \times 0.016]$
Corrected total calcium: $[0.8 \times (\text{normal albumin} - \text{measured albumin})] + Ca$

Bodywater deficit : $\dfrac{0.6 \times \text{weight (kg)} \times (\text{patient Na} - \text{normal Na})}{\text{normal Na}}$

Aa gradient: $[(713 \times FIO_2) - (PaCO_2/0.8)] - PaO_2 = 150 - (PaCO_2/0.8)] - PaO_2$
Anion gap: $Na - Cl + HCO_3$ (normal value is between 8 and 12 mEq/L)
MAP (mean arterial pressure): diastolic BP + [(systolic BP − diastolic BP)/3]
Cerebral perfusion pressure: MAP − ICP (intracranial pressure)

## Statistics

Incidence: Number of **new cases** of a disease in a population in a certain period of time

Prevalence: Number of **existing cases** of a disease in a population at a specific time point

Sensitivity: This determines how well the test is able to detect disease.

$$\frac{\text{Number of patients with disease and positive test}}{\text{Total number with disease}}$$

Specificity: This determines how well the test detects the absence of disease.

$$\frac{\text{Number of patients without disease and negative test}}{\text{Total number without disease}}$$

Relative risk : $\dfrac{\text{Incidence in exposed}}{\text{Incidence in unexposed}}$

Positive predictive value (PPV): Test precision or the probability that a patient truly has the disease when they test positive. Calculation: true positive/all positive.

Negative predictive value (NPV): Probability that a patient truly does **not** have the disease when they test negative. Increased sensitivity increases NPV, and the lower the prevalence of a disease, the higher the NPV. Calculation: true negative/all negative.

True positive: Patient **with** disease and positive test

False positive: Patient **without** disease and positive test

True negative: Patient **without** disease and negative test

False negative:  Patient **with** disease and negative test

|  | **With Disease** | **Without Disease** |
| --- | --- | --- |
| Positive Test | True Positive (A) | False Positive (B) |
| Negative Test | False Negative (C) | True Negative (D) |

Sensitivity: A/A+C

Specificity: D/B+D

PPV: A/A+B

NPV: D/D+C

Relative risk: [A/(A+B)]/[C/(C+D)]
Odds ratio: AxD/CxB

Absolute risk: (incidence of disease in exposed) − (incidence of disease in unexposed)

Number needed to treat (NNT): Number of patients that need to be treated in order to prevent one negative outcome. Calculation: 1/absolute risk

Length time bias: Screening tests will tend to be able to detect cases of slowly progressive disease much better than rapidly progressive diseases, just because of the nature of having a longer asymptomatic period

Lead time bias: Screening tests detects disease before symptomatic phase, increasing the time between diagnosis and death.

Likelihood ratio: true positive/false positive

Null hypothesis: The statement that the thing being tested is **not** associated with the outcome

Type I error ($\alpha$): probability of detecting a difference when one does not actually exist (for example concluding that a drug works when it actually does not)

Type II error ($\beta$): Probability of **not** detecting a difference when on does actually exist (for example concluding that a drug does **not** work when it actually does)

Power: Probability of **NOT** detecting a difference when one actually does **not** exist (eg, concluding that a drug does **NOT** work and it actually does NOT work). Power is increase by larger sample size.

Calculation: 1 – type II error

$p$ value: probability that the results of a study could happen by chance alone. Generally $p < 0.05$ is considered statistically significant.

Precision (reliability): reproducibility of the results of a test

Validity (accuracy): whether the test actually correctly measures what it is trying to measure

## Study Types

Randomized controlled: Subjects are blindly assigned to groups being studied. (Eg, if you are studying a cholesterol drug, patients are randomly assigned to the treatment group and placebo group.)

Cohort study: Exposed subject are identified and followed for a certain time to study disease outcome.

Case-control study: Identify cases and non-cases and studied retrospectively to find possible risk factors.

## Experimental Errors

Recall bias: Overestimation or underestimation of risk factors due to the fact that patients may not recall accurately. Relevant to retrospective studies.

Interviewer bias: Interpretation of data being skewed due to the scientist's personal bias. This occurs when the study is not a blinded study.

Unacceptability bias: Patients may not report certain information because they feel ashamed or want to please the scientist.

# CHAPTER 1

# The Basics

## QUICK RADIOLOGY

### Chest X-ray

What is the first thing that you should check when evaluating a radiographic study?

Check the name of the patient as well as the date and medical record number.

How can you determine if the chest x-ray (CXR) is adequate?

1. Penetration: Disk spaces can be seen without distinguishing the details of the spine.
2. Inspiratory effort: Diaphragm anteriorly should be below rib 7.
3. Rotation: Spinous processes of thoracic vertebrae should be midway between clavicles.

What is a posterior-anterior (PA) film?

Posterior-anterior film: The x-ray is shot from the back of the patient to the plate in front of the patient.

What is an anterior-posterior (AP) film?

Anterior-posterior film: The x-ray is shot from the front of the patient to the back of the patient.

When is an AP film appropriate?

When a patient is bed bound

How is the image altered in an AP film?

The heart appears large.

How should you approach reading a CXR?

Remember **A, B, C, D plus lungs and soft tissue**

**Airway:** Trachea should be midline.

**Bones:** Check for any bony defects, fractures, osteolytic lesions.

**Cardiac:** The heart should be less than ½ the width of the chest.

**Diaphragm:** There should be no blunting of the costophrenic angles.

No free air should be seen under the hemidiaphragm.

**Lungs:** Look for any nodules, opacification, bronchial markings.

**Soft tissue:** Look for any lesions, lymphadenopathy, masses.

What structure does each of the following types of infiltrates obscure?

Right middle lobe

Right lower lobe

Left upper lobe

Left lower lobe

Right atrium

Right diaphragmatic border

Left heart border

Left diaphragmatic border

What classic features are seen on a chest x-ray with congestive heart failure?

Cephalization of vessels; **curly B lines**

Name the parts of the CXR shown below?

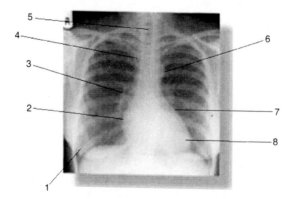

(Reproduced, with permission, from William Herring, MD, FACR; Radiology Residency Program Director at Albert Einstein Medical Center in Philadelphia, PA. Available at: http://www.learningradiology.com)

1. Sharp costophrenic angle
2. Right atrium
3. Hilum and main bronchus
4. Superior vena cava
5. Trachea (midline)
6. Aortic arch
7. Left atrium
8. Left ventricle

## Other Radiologic Studies

What is a kidneys, ureter, and bladder (KUB)?

X-ray which looks at the kidney, ureter, and bladder

What structures do computed tomographic (CT) scans visualize best?

CT scans visualize bone best and can identify acute bleeds.

What structures does a magnetic resonance imaging (MRI) visualize best?

Soft tissue

Name the radiographic study you would use to evaluate each of the following:

Biliary tract

Right upper quadrant ultrasound

Differentiate between loculated and unloculated pleural effusion

Lateral decubitus film—fluid that is loculated will not layer out

Carotid artery stenosis

Carotid ultrasound

Kidney stones

KUB

Stroke

MRI of the brain; CT to rule out hemorrhage

Anterior cruciate ligament (ACL) tear of the knee

MRI of the knee

Acute cholecystitis

Hepatobiliary iminodiacetic acid (HIDA) scan

Name what each of the following
radiographic findings is most
commonly indicative of:

| | |
|---|---|
| Flattened diaphragms | Chronic obstructive pulmonary disease (COPD) |
| Blunted costophrenic angles | Pleural effusion |
| Air outside pleural lines | Pneumothorax |
| Consolidation of lung parenchyma | Pneumonia |
| Dilated loops of small bowel | Small bowel obstruction |
| Air fluid levels | Small bowel obstruction |

## QUICK EKG INTERPRETATION

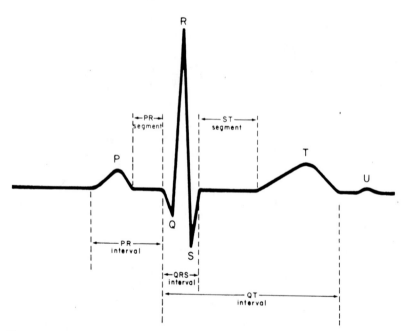

**Figure 1-1**   Parts of the EKG. (*Reproduced, with permission, from Tintinalli JE. Emergency Medicine: A comprehensive study guide. 6th ed. New York: McGraw-Hill, 2004:181.*)

**Step 1:** Calculate the rate (Fig 1-2).
Rate = beats per minute.
The easy way to calculate the rate is **300/(# big boxes between two QRS complexes) or 300, 150, 100, 75, 60, 50.**
300/3 = 100.
In this example, the rate is about 100 beats per minute.

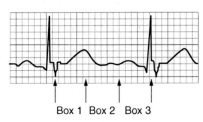

Box 1   Box 2   Box 3

**Figure 1-2**    Rate calculation example. In
this EKG, the rate is 300/3 = 100 beats/min.

**Step 2:** Calculate the rhythm (Fig 1-3).
Ask the question: Is there a P wave before each QRS? And, are the P waves of the same morphology? If yes, then the rhythm is sinus.
In the example, there is a P wave of the same morphology before each QRS, which indicates that the patient is in sinus rhythm. If there were a lack of P waves or a disorganized rhythm, a differential diagnosis, which you will find in Chapter 2, would come into play.

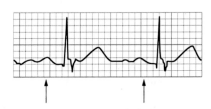

**Figure 1-3**    Sinus rhythm.

**Step 3:** Determine the axis (Fig 1-4).
Rules of thumb:
If I and aVF are positive, then axis is normal.
If I is positive and aVF is negative, check lead II.
If lead II is positive, then the axis is normal.

If lead II is negative, then there is left axis deviation.
If I is negative and aVF is positive, then there is right axis deviation.

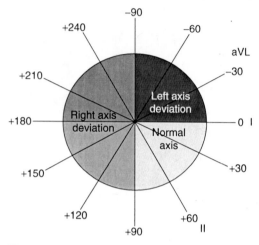

**Figure 1-4**

**Step 4:** Evaluate the intervals.
One large box = 0.20 seconds.
One small box = 0.04 seconds.
Normal measurements:
P wave <0.12 seconds
PR interval (beginning of P wave to beginning of QRS complex) 0.12-0.2 seconds
QRS interval (beginning of the Q to the end of the S wave) <0.12 seconds
QT interval (beginning of QRS to the end of the T wave) 0.33-0.47 seconds

If PR <0.12, **then** junctional rhythm or bypass tract
If PR >0.2, **then** atrioventricular (AV) block
If QRS >0.12, **then** either a left bundle branch block (LBBB), right bundle branch block (RBBB), **or** a nonspecific conduction delay

**Step 5:** Check for hypertrophy.
*Atrial hypertrophy*

**Right atrium:** tall P waves in II, III, and aVF or $V_1$ or $V_2$
**Left atrium:** notched P waves in limb leads
*Ventricular hypertrophy*
**Left ventricular hypertrophy:** height of S (mm) in $V_1$ + height of R (mm) in $V_5$ >35 mm
**Right ventricular hypertrophy:** height of R (mm)/height of S (mm) in V1 >1

**Step 6:** Look for ischemic changes.
ST elevation or depression
T-wave inversion

**Q waves indicating old infarct**

# PREVENTATIVE MEDICINE

## Adult Immunizations

**Table 1-1** Adult Immunization Recommendations

| | |
|---|---|
| Tdap (tetanus toxoid, reduced diphtheria toxoid, acellular pertussis) | Give complete series if patient has not received it.<br>Age 19-65 as a booster every 10 years instead of Td.<br>Especially important with outbreak of pertussis. |
| Influenza | Annually. Can be given to all patients but especially those with immunocompromised states, such as pregnant women, chronic disease states.<br>FluMist nasal spray can only be used in "healthy" people aged 2-49 who are not pregnant. |
| Pneumococcal | Patients aged >65<br>Patients aged >50 with chronic diseases or immunocompromised<br>Booster if aged >65 and primary vaccine >5 years ago |
| Varicella | Patients with no history of disease and/or negative titers. Two doses 1-2 months apart. |
| MMR (measles, mumps, rubella) | Born after 1957 and never immunized. Two doses at least 1 month apart. |
| HBV (hepatitis B vaccine) | Not previously immunized and at increased risk of exposure such as occupational and social exposure |

## PREVENTATIVE SCREENING

**Table 1-2** Preventative Screening Recommendations

| Condition | Recommendation |
|---|---|
| Abdominal aortic aneurysm | **Men aged 65-75** who have smoking history; **one time** screening by ultrasound |
| Blood pressure | Men and women aged >18; every 2 years |
| Breast cancer | Women **aged ≥40; every 1 to 2 years.** If there is a family history of a first-degree relative, then screen 10 years before the age at which the cancer was detected. Typically by mammography. |
| Cervical cancer | Women starting at age 21 using a Pap smear cytologic test. Women aged 21-29 screen with Pap smear cytologic test every 2 years unless there is an abnormality detected, then follow the specific guidelines.  Women aged ≥30-65 screen with Pap smear cytologic test  + HPV screening every 3 years if they have had 3 consecutive normal Pap tests. Stop screening at 65-70 years of age if 3 or more consecutive normal Pap test and no abnormals in the last 10 years. |
| *Chlamydia* infection | Sexually active women aged ≤25 and other women at increased risk |
| Cholesterol screening | Patients at high risk for CAD, initial screening: men aged 20-35 and women aged ≥20. Otherwise: all men aged ≥35 and all women aged ≥45 every 5 years. Using fasting lipid profile or non-fasting total cholesterol and HDL |
| Colorectal cancer | Men and women **aged >50 to 75**. Annual fecal occult blood test and sigmoidoscopy every 5 years *or* **colonoscopy every 10 years**. Screening to be started earlier if patient at high risk. |
| Diabetes, type II | Asymptomatic men and women with blood pressure >135/80 |
| *Gonorrhea* infection | Sexually active women aged ≤25 and other women at increased risk |
| HIV | All adults and adolescents at increased risk for infection. *All* pregnant women. |
| Osteoporosis | Postmenopausal **women aged ≥65** and women aged ≥60 who are at high risk for osteoporotic fractures. DEXA scan is used. |
| Ovarian cancer | Routine screening is *not recommended*. |

*(Continued)*

**Table 1-2** Preventative Screening Recommendations (Continued)

| Condition | Recommendation |
|---|---|
| Prostate cancer | USPSTF has found insufficient evidence for or against screening using digital rectal examination or serum PSA, but most physicians consider screening men between the age of 40 and 75. |
| Syphilis infection | Men and women at increased risk and *all* pregnant women. |

DEXA, dual energy x-ray absorptiometry; HDL, high-density lipoprotein; PSA, prostate-specific antigen.

# FLUIDS AND ELECTROLYTES

## Fluids

| | |
|---|---|
| What percentage of body mass is water? | 50% to 70% |
| In what two compartments is body water stored and what is the portion in each? | Intracellular ($2/3$)<br>Extracellular ($1/3$) |
| How is extracellular fluid separated? | Intravascular ($1/4$); extravascular or interstitial ($3/4$) |
| What percentage of body mass does intracellular water account for? | 40% |
| What percentage of body mass does extracellular water account for? | 20% |
| What percentage of body mass does blood account for? | About 7% |
| What physical examination signs can be used to assess volume status? | Skin turgor, mucous membranes, pulse, urine output, acute weight change |

| | |
|---|---|
| What are signs of hypovolemia? | Tachycardia, tachypnea, dry mucous membranes, decreased urine output, decreased blood pressure, decreased skin turgor |
| What is normal urine output in an adult? | Above 30 cc/h; on average 0.5-1 cc/kg/h |
| How do you calculate maintenance fluids per hour? | 4/2/1 rule: 4 mL/kg (up to 10 kg); 2 mL/kg(from 11 to 30 kg); 1 mL/kg (>30 kg) |
| How do you calculate maintenance fluids per day? | 100/50/20 rule: 100 mL/kg (up to 10 kg); 50 mL/kg (from 11 to 30 kg); 20 mL/kg (>30 kg) |
| What are each of the following IV fluids comprised of? | |
| D5W | 5% dextrose in water |
| D10W | 10% dextrose in water |
| Normal saline (NS) | 154 mEq Na, 154 mEq Cl |
| ½ NS | 77 mEq Na, 77 mEq Cl |
| ¼ NS | 39 mEq Na, 39 mEq Cl |
| Lactated Ringer | 130 mEq Na, 110 mEq Cl, 4 mEq K, 3 mEq Ca, 28 mEq lactate |
| What are the two most commonly used maintenance fluids? | D5 ½ NS or D5 ½ NS with 20 mEq K |
| What type of IV fluids should be given for fluid resuscitation? | NS or lactated Ringer because they are isotonic |

# Electrolytes

*Hyperkalemia*

| | |
|---|---|
| What is the normal range for potassium? | 3.5-5.0 mEq/L |
| What are the causes of hyperkalemia? | Increased load vs decreased excretion: **Increased load:** exogenous $K^+$ ingestion, blood transfusion, tissue injury (rhabdomyolysis, burns), acidosis, hypoaldosteronism **Decreased excretion:** renal failure, $K^+$-sparing diuretics |

**What is pseudohyperkalemia?**

Elevated $K^+$ in a blood sample due to hemolysis

**What are the signs and symptoms?**

Muscle weakness, paresthesias, areflexia, bradycardia, respiratory failure, EKG changes

**What are the characteristic EKG findings?**

**Peaked T waves**

Prolonged PR interval, widening of QRS, P-wave loss, (Fig 1-5)

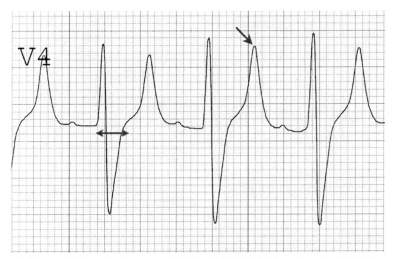

**Figure 1-5**  Peaked T waves (arrow), widened QRS (double arrow), and subtle flattening of the P waves are seen in this patient with a serum K of 7.1. *(Reproduced, with permission, from Knoop KJ, Stack LB, Storrow AB, et al.* Atlas of Emergency Medicine. *3rd ed. New York: McGraw-Hill; 2010:778.)*

**Above what level are symptoms usually seen?**

$K^+ > 6.5$.

**How is hyperkalemia treated?**

1. Protect cells by increasing membrane threshold: calcium gluconate (cardioprotective)
2. Drive $K^+$ into cells: sodium bicarbonate, insulin with glucose
3. Excrete $K^+$: kayexalate (binds $K^+$), furosemide, dialysis

**What is the mnemonic for treatment of hyperkalemia?**

C BIG K Drop:

Calcium gluconate

Bicarbonate

Insulin

Glucose

Kayexalate

Dialysis

r

o

p

**What acid-base disturbance can lead to hyperkalemia?**

Acidosis

*Hypokalemia*

**What are some causes of hypokalemia?**

Vomiting, diarrhea, nasogastric (NG) tube suction, diuretic use (thiazides are a common culprit), insulin, amphotericin, hypomagnesemia

**What are the signs and symptoms of hypokalemia?**

Nausea, vomiting, weakness, paresthesias, hyporeflexia, ileus, digoxin sensitivity, v-tach, and EKG changes

**What acid-base disturbance can cause hypokalemia?**

Alkalosis

**What are the characteristic EKG findings of hypokalemia?**

T-wave depression, U waves, prolonged QT and ST depression (Fig 1-6)

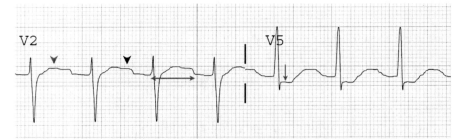

**Figure 1-6**   This EKG demonstrates multiple findings consistent with hypokalemia: flattened T waves (gray arrowhead), U waves (black arrowhead), prolonged QT (QU) intervals (double arrow), and ST-segment depression (arrow). This patient's potassium level was 1.9. *(Reproduced, with permission, from Knoop KJ, Stack LB, Storrow AB, et al. Atlas of Emergency Medicine. 3rd ed. New York: McGraw-Hill; 2010:777.)*

| | |
|---|---|
| **How is severe hypokalemia acutely treated?** | IV KCl |
| **What is the major side effect of IV potassium?** | Burning sensation at IV site through which it is being administered |
| **How can the burning be avoided when administering IV potassium?** | Slow infusion usually not more than 10 mEq/h |
| **How can mild or chronic hypokalemia be treated?** | Oral KCl supplementation or potassium-rich foods |
| **What electrolyte level should be checked in a patient with hypokalemia?** | Magnesium; hypomagnesemia can precipitate hypokalemia. |
| **What medication can be used to treat hypokalemia?** | Potassium-sparing diuretic (eg, spironolactone) |

## Hypercalcemia

**What is the normal range for calcium?**  9.0-10.6 (serum calcium)

**What are the causes for hypercalcemia?**  Mnemonics **CHIMPANZEES:**
Calcium supplementation
Hyperparathyroidism
Iatrogenic
Milk alkali syndrome
Paget disease
Addison disease
Neoplasm
Zollinger-Ellison syndrome (MEN I)
Excess vitamin A
Excess vitamin D
Sarcoidosis

**What is a common iatrogenic cause of hypercalcemia?**  Thiazide diuretics

**What are the symptoms of hypercalcemia?**  **Stones** (kidney stones), **bones** (bone pain), **abdominal groans** (abdominal pain, nausea, constipation), and **psychiatric overtones** (confusion, concentration, fatigue)

**What does the EKG look like?**  Prolonged **PR** interval, short QT interval

**What is the treatment?**  IV hydration, loop diuretic (furosemide)

**How is it treated in refractory cases?**  Calcitonin, pamidronate, etidronate, glucocorticoids, plicamycin, dialysis

## Hypocalcemia

**What are the causes of hypocalcemia?**  Renal failure, vitamin D deficiency, pancreatitis, diuretics, hypomagnesemia, parathyroidectomy

**What can cause a pseudohypocalcemia?**  Hypoalbuminemia

How can the true calcium level be calculated in hypoalbuminemia?

$0.8 \times (4 -$ plasma albumin level) $+$ calcium level $=$ true calcium level

What are the two classic signs of hypocalcemia?

**Trousseau** and **Chvostek** signs

What is Trousseau sign?

Carpal spasm with arterial occlusion using a blood pressure cuff

What is Chvostek sign?

Facial spasm with tapping of the facial nerve

What are some other signs and symptoms of hypocalcemia?

Tetany, seizures, perioral paresthesias, altered mental status, fatigue, weakness, EKG changes, abdominal cramping, convulsions

What is the classic EKG finding with hypocalcemia?

**Prolonged QT interval**

What is the treatment for acute hypocalcemia?

IV calcium gluconate

What is the treatment for chronic hypocalcemia?

Vitamin D with oral calcium tablets

*Hypernatremia*

What is the normal range for sodium?

135-145 mEq/L

What are the causes of hypernatremia?

**Hypovolemia:** decreased oral intake of water secondary to illness or altered mental status; increased water loss such as diuresis, vomiting, diarrhea, hyperaldosteronism

**Hypervolemia:** hypertonic fluid administration, excess ingestion of salt, Cushing syndrome, Conn syndrome

**Isovolemia:** diabetes insipidus, skin loss

**How do you calculate water deficit in hypernatremia?**

$0.6 \times$ weight (kg) $\times$ (measured Na/ normal Na) $- 1$

**What are the signs and symptoms of hypernatremia?**

Seizure, coma, ataxia, lethargy, irritability, spasticity, edema

**What is the treatment for hypernatremia?**

Treatment is dependent on each of the following underlying causea of hypernatremia:

**Hypovolemia:** Replace fluid with isotonic saline. Replace ½ of water deficit in first 24 hours and ½ over the next 48-72 hours.

**Hypervolemia:** Loop diuretics to increase sodium excretion and fluid replacement with ½ NS

**Isovolemia:** Fluid replacement with ½ NS (½ water deficit in first 24 hours and ½ over next 48-72 hours). If patient has central diabetes insipidus, give vasopressin.

**What is the risk of rapid correction of hypernatremia?**

Cerebral edema
CENTRAL PONTINE MYELINOLYSIS ?
HIGH + LOW NE?

**What is the maximum rate at which plasma osmolality can be corrected?**

2 mOsm/kg/h

**What is the maximum rate at which sodium concentration can be corrected safely?**

1 mEq/L/h
(0.5/hr IS BETTER)

*Hyponatremia*

**What is the differential diagnosis of hyponatremia?**    See Fig 1-7.

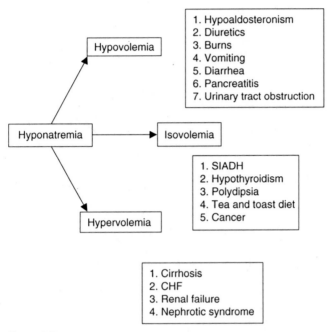

**Figure 1-7**

**What is pseudohyponatremia?**    There is no true sodium deficit, but appears to be because the serum is occupied by lipids or protein.

**What is factitious hyponatremia?**    Normal total body sodium but decreased serum sodium because of an osmotic flow of water into serum secondary to excess glucose or mannitol in the serum

**How is serum osmolality calculated?**    $2 \times$ Na + blood urea nitrogen (BUN)/2.8 + glucose/18

**How is hyponatremia evaluated?**          See Fig 1-8.

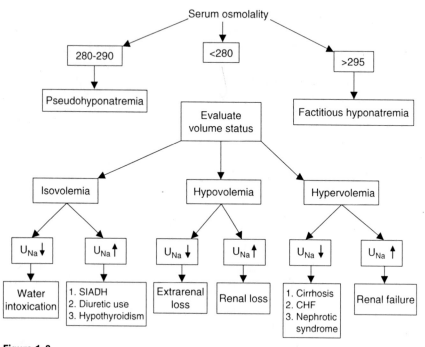

**Figure 1-8**

| | |
|---|---|
| **What are the signs and symptoms of hyponatremia?** | Seizure, coma, lethargy, weakness, nausea, vomiting, ileus, altered mental status |
| **What is the treatment for hypotonic hypovolemic hyponatremia?** | Correct the underlying disorder and fluid resuscitation with IV normal saline (NS). |
| **What is the treatment for hypotonic hypervolemic hyponatremia?** | Fluid restriction. Diuretics like furosemide are helpful. |
| **What is the treatment for hypotonic isovolemic hyponatremia?** | Treat the underlying cause. Fluid restriction. |
| **What is the maximum speed at which hyponatremia can be safely corrected?** | 1 mEq/h |
| **What can happen if sodium is corrected too quickly?** | Central pontine myelinolysis |

*Hyperphosphatemia*

| | |
|---|---|
| **What is the normal range of phosphate?** | 2.5-4.5 mg/dL |
| **What are the most common causes of hyperphosphatemia?** | Iatrogenic |
| **What are other causes of hyperphosphatemia?** | Hypoparathyroidism, hypocalcemia, renal failure, rhabdomyolysis, tumor lysis |
| **What are the signs and symptoms of hyperphosphatemia?** | Heart block, ectopic soft tissue calcification |
| **What is the treatment for hyperphosphatemia?** | Aluminum hydroxide; sevelamer hydrochloride (Renagel); calcium acetate (Phoslo); lanthanum carbonate (Fosrenol); insulin and glucose; in severe cases—dialysis |

*Hypophosphatemia*

| | |
|---|---|
| **What are the causes of hypophosphatemia?** | Hyperparathyroidism, diuresis, decreased po (oral) intake, renal tubular acidosis, hypokalemia, hypomagnesemia, acetazolamide, glucose, and insulin |
| **What are the signs and symptoms of hypophosphatemia?** | Proximal muscle weakness, ataxia, rhabdomyolysis, paresthesias, hemolytic anemia, seizure |
| **What is the treatment for hypophosphatemia?** | Potassium phosphate of sodium phosphate supplementation |

*Hypermagnesemia*

| | |
|---|---|
| **What is the normal range of magnesium?** | 1.5-2.5 mEq/L |
| **What are the causes of hypermagnesemia?** | Iatrogenic, renal failure, tumor lysis |
| **What are the signs and symptoms of hypermagnesemia?** | Weakness, fatigue, ↓ deep tendon reflexes, hypotension, paresthesias, coma, decreased respirations |

**What is the treatment for hypermagnesemia?**

Calcium gluconate and dialysis in refractory cases

## Hypomagnesemia

**What are the causes of hypomagnesemia?**

Malabsorption, diarrhea, vomiting, NG tube suction, alcoholic patient, diuresis, hypokalemia or hypocalciuria induce hypomagnesemia, insulin and glucose administration, short bowel syndrome, total parenteral nutrition, hypercalcemia

**What are the signs and symptoms of hypomagnesemia?**

Weakness, hyperreflexia, seizure, altered mental status, torsades de pointes, atrial fibrillation, hypokalemia, and hypocalcemia refractory to replacement

**What EKG changes would you expect to see in a patient with hypomagnesemia?**

Prolonged QT and PR intervals, flattened T waves; may see torsades de pointes

**What is the treatment for hypomagnesemia?**

Magnesium sulfate IV

**What other electrolyte abnormalities are related to hypomagnesemia?**

Hypokalemia and hypocalcemia—if magnesium is low, these electrolyte abnormalities become refractory to treatment.

**Name the electrolyte abnormality associated with the following EKG (Fig. 1-9).**

Hyperkalemia with peaked T waves

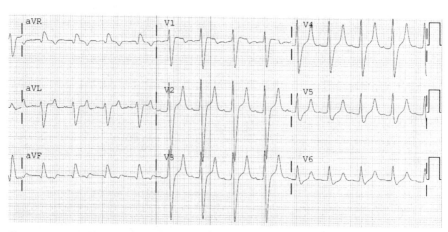

**Figure 1-9** Peaked T waves. *(Reproduced, with permission, from Knoop KJ, Stack LB, Storrow AB, et al. Atlas of Emergency Medicine. 3rd ed. New York: McGraw-Hill, 2010: 778. Photo contributor: R. Jason Thurman, MD.)*

# NUTRITION

Name the type of diet you would order
for each of the following types of
patients:

| | |
|---|---|
| Patients who have no dietary restrictions | Regular diet |
| Patients with diabetes type I or II | Diabetic diet or American Diabetes Association (ADA) diet; be sure to specify the number of calories per day |
| Patients with renal failure or liver disorders | Protein-restricted diet; specify the amount of protein per day |
| Patients who do not have teeth or have difficulty with chewing and/or swallowing | Mechanical soft or pureed food |
| Patients with pancreatitis | Npo (nothing by mouth) |
| Patients who are at risk for aspiration | Npo |
| Patients with coronary artery disease | Low-fat diet; cardiac diet |
| Patients who are being transitioned from npo to an oral diet | Clear liquids (includes clear broth, gelatin), then full liquids |
| Patients with syndrome of inappropriate secretion of antidiuretic hormone (SIADH) | Fluid-restricted diet; specify the amount of fluid per day |
| Normally, what is the daily protein requirement for an adult? | 1 g/kg per 24 hours |
| Normally, what is the daily carbohydrate requirement for an adult? | 35 kcal/kg per 24 hours |
| How many kilocalories (kcal) in 1 g of fat? | 9 kcal |
| How many kcal in 1 g of carbohydrate? | 4 kcal |
| How many kcal in 1 g of protein? | 4 kcal |
| What lab test is used to determine chronic nutritional status? | Albumin, since the half-life is about 20 days |
| What lab test is used to determine acute nutritional change? | Prealbumin, since the half-life is about 3 days |
| Name the fat-soluble vitamins. | D, E, A, K (DEAK) |

| | |
|---|---|
| Where are the fat-soluble vitamins absorbed? | In the terminal ileum |
| Where is vitamin $B_{12}$ absorbed? | In the terminal ileum |
| What must bind $B_{12}$ in order for it to be absorbed? | Intrinsic factor |
| Where is iron absorbed? | Jejunum |
| Where is intrinsic factor produced? | It is produced by the gastric parietal cells. |

Name the effect on the body with each of the following deficiencies:

| | |
|---|---|
| Vitamin $B_1$ deficiency | Beriberi, Wernike-Korsakoff syndrome |
| Vitamin $B_2$ deficiency | Cheilosis |
| Vitamin $B_3$ deficiency | Pellagra |
| Vitamin $B_6$ deficiency | Associated with isoniazid (INH) use |
| Vitamin $B_{12}$ deficiency | Megaloblastic anemia, neurologic symptoms |
| Zinc deficiency | Poor wound healing, dermatitis, alopecia |
| Folic acid deficiency | Megaloblastic anemia |
| Vitamin C deficiency | Bleeding gums, scurvy |
| Vitamin A deficiency | Poor wound healing |
| Vitamin K deficiency | Bleeding, elevated PT and PTT |

| | |
|---|---|
| What are the vitamin K-dependent clotting factors? | Factors 2, 7, 9, 10 |
| What is TPN? | Total parenteral nutrition |
| What are the indications for TPN use? | Npo for >7 days |
| | Pancreatitis |
| | Anorexia |
| | Enterocutaneous fistula |
| | Ileus that is not resolving |
| | Burn patients |
| | Patients unable to take food by mouth |

| | |
|---|---|
| What are the three main components of TPN? | 1. Amino acids<br>2. Dextrose<br>3. Fat |
| What percentage of TPN is fat? | 10% (20% in the form of intralipid) |
| What percentage of TPN calories comes from dextrose? | 50% to 70% |
| What percentage of total calories comes from fat? | 30% to 50% |
| What percentage of total calories comes from amino acids (or protein)? | 10% to 20% |
| How is basal energy expenditure (BEE) calculated in a male? | $66 + (13.7 \times$ weight [kg]$) + (5 \times$ height [cm]$) - (6.8 \times$ age$)$ |
| How is BEE calculated in a female? | $65 + (9.6 \times$ weight [kg]$) + (1.8 \times$ height [cm]$) - (4.7 \times$ age$)$ |
| What are the complications of TPN? | Fatty liver, acalculous cholecystitis, hyperosmolality, line infection, refeeding syndrome, cholestasis |
| What is refeeding syndrome? | Low potassium, phosphate, and magnesium after refeeding of a patient who was previously starving |
| What is PPN? | Partial parenteral nutrition |
| When would PPN be used? | In patients who can tolerate some nutrition orally and only need some supplementation |
| A patient who becomes jaundiced while on TPN or PPN most likely has what condition? | Cholestasis |

## BLOOD PRODUCTS AND TRANSFUSIONS

| | |
|---|---|
| What blood products are measured when checking a complete blood count (CBC)? | White blood cells, hemoglobin, hematocrit, platelets, red blood cells |

Name the blood products described below:

| | |
|---|---|
| Contains no platelets or clotting factors | Packed red blood cells (PRBC) |
| Contains red blood cell (RBC), white blood cells (WBC), plasma, and platelets and can be used for an acute, heavy bleed | Whole blood |
| Used to replace clotting factors | Fresh frozen plasma (FFP) |
| Contains von Willebrand factor, factors VIII and XIII, and fibrinogen. Used in hemophilia A, fibrinogen deficiency, and von Willebrand disease. | Cryoprecipitate |
| Used to replace low platelets | Platelets |

Name the blood tests described below:

| | |
|---|---|
| Tests the intrinsic coagulation pathway | Partial thromboplastin time (PTT) |
| Tests the extrinsic coagulation pathway | Prothrombin time (PT) |
| Measures PT | International normalized ratio (INR) |

| | |
|---|---|
| What is the problem with using FFP in patients on Coumadin? | It will reverse the anticoagulation quickly; however, it is more difficult to get the patient back to a therapeutic level. |
| What else can be used to reverse anticoagulation in a patient on Coumadin? | Vitamin K, but much slower than FFP |
| Which foods have vitamin K? | Leafy green vegetables |
| What is involved in normal coagulation? | Damage to the endothelium leads to platelet binding and aggregation; coagulation factors then help lay down fibrin to form and stabilize a clot. |

What is a therapeutic INR level for a patient on Coumadin for each of the following underlying conditions:

| | |
|---|---|
| Atrial fibrillation | INR 2-3 |
| Mechanical prosthetic heart valve | INR 2.5-3.5 |
| Deep venous thrombosis (DVT) | INR 2-3 |
| Recurrent thromboembolic events with therapeutic INR | INR 2.5-3.5 |

When should you consider a blood transfusion in a normal, healthy patient?

When hemoglobin drops below 8

When should you consider a blood transfusion in a patient with coronary artery disease?

When hemoglobin drops below 10

How does 1 U of PRBC affect the hemoglobin and hematocrit?

1 U should increase the hemoglobin by 1 g/dL and hematocrit by 3%.

What is the formula for converting hematocrit to hemoglobin?

Hematocrit $\div$ 3 = hemoglobin.

What study should be ordered if you are considering transfusing a patient?

Type and cross

What is a type and cross?

The patient's RBCs are cross-matched to available donor blood for transfusion. In this process, the patient's serum is checked for preformed antibodies to the RBCs of the donor.

What is a type and screen?

The patient's blood type and Rh antigen are determined and the donor's blood is screened for common antibodies.

What blood type is considered the universal donor?

O

What blood type is considered the universal recipient?

AB

What are the two main complications of a blood transfusion that a patient should know about before consenting for a transfusion?

Possibility of acquiring an infectious disease and possibility of rejection

What is the most common cause of rejection during a blood transfusion?

Clerical error leading to ABO incompatibility

What are the most common signs and symptoms seen of an acute rejection?

Fever, chills, tachycardia, shock, acute renal failure

What is the treatment of a rejection to a blood transfusion?

*Stop the transfusion!* IV fluid resuscitation and make sure the patient has good urine output. If urine output is not sufficient, furosemide (Lasix) can be administered.

After a transfusion, what would you expect to happen to the ionized calcium in the blood?

It decreases because of the preservative citrate used to store blood.

What is the most common transfusion-related infection?

Hepatitis

What is the risk of infection with hepatitis B from a blood transfusion?

1 in 200,000 U of blood

What is the risk of infection with hepatitis C from a blood transfusion?

1 in 2 million U of blood

What is the risk of getting infected with human immunodeficiency virus (HIV) from a blood transfusion?

1 in 2 million U of blood

How long can PRBCs be stored?

6 weeks

What is the life span of a RBC?

120 days

What is thrombocytopenia?

Platelet count <200,000

At what platelet count is there a risk for spontaneous intercranial bleeding?

Platelet count <20,000

In an actively bleeding patient or a patient who is preoperative, what should the platelet count be?

A minimum of 50,000

In what cases of thrombocytopenia are platelets not transfused?

Do not transfuse platelets in patients with thrombotic thrombocytopenic purpura (TTP), idiopathic thrombocytopenic purpura (ITP), and disseminated intravascular coagulation (DIC), because platelet transfusion will only perpetuate the problem. Platelets are only transfused if the patient is actively bleeding.

# CHAPTER 2

# Cardiology

## HYPERTENSION

| | |
|---|---|
| How is hypertension defined? | Prehypertension: 120-139/80-89<br>Stage 1: 140-159/90-99<br>Stage 2: >160/>100 |
| What is the most common cause of hypertension? | 90% is essential or idiopathic. |
| What are some secondary causes of hypertension? | 1. Cardiovascular: coarctation of aorta, aortic regurgitation<br>2. Renal: renal artery stenosis, polycystic kidney disease, glomerular disease<br>3. Endocrine: eclampsia, pheochromocytoma, primary hyperaldosteronism (Cushing and Conn) |
| When would you suspect a possible secondary cause? | Resistant hypertension despite multiple medications, diagnosis of hypertension at age <25 or >55 |
| Define hypertensive urgency. | Systolic >180, diastolic >120 **with *no* end-organ failure** |
| Define hypertensive emergency. | Also known as malignant hypertension; systolic >180, diastolic >120; ***with* end-organ failure** |
| What are the signs and symptoms of malignant hypertension? | 1. Change in mental status<br>2. Papilledema<br>3. Anuria (sign of renal failure)<br>4. Heart failure<br>5. New-onset neurologic change |

What is the treatment for malignant hypertension?

Nitroprusside or nitroglycerine

In malignant hypertension, by how much should the blood pressure be reduced in 1 hour?

**Do not** decrease by more than ¼ within 2-6 hours, otherwise the patient will be at risk for a stroke.

How do you calculate mean arterial pressure (MAP)?

$(2 \times \text{diastolic} + \text{systolic})/3$

What hypertensive treatment is favorable for a patient with each of the following comorbidities?

   No comorbidities

If they fail lifestyle modification for 6 months, add a thiazide diuretic.

   Postmyocardial infarction (MI)

Beta-blocker and angiotensin-converting enzyme (ACE) inhibitor

   Benign prostatic hyperplasia (BPH)

Alpha-blocker

   Congestive heart failure (CHF)

ACE inhibitor

   Osteoporosis

Thiazide diuretics (do not excrete calcium)

   Diabetes

ACE inhibitor

   African American

Calcium channel blocker, diuretic

What are the relative contraindications for each of the following treatments?

   ACE inhibitors

Teratogenic in pregnancy, in renal artery stenosis, renal failure

   Beta-blocker

Chronic obstructive pulmonary disease (COPD), asthma, diabetes, hyperkalemia

   Short-acting calcium channel blockers

Prior MI, CHF

   Potassium (K)-sparing diuretics

Renal failure (can lead to hyperkalemia)

   Thiazide diuretics

Diabetes (can cause hyperglycemia)

What are the most common side effects for each of the following treatments?

| | |
|---|---|
| ACE inhibitors | Cough, angioedema, hyperkalemia |
| Beta-blockers | Bronchospasm, bradycardia, fatigue |
| Alpha-blockers | Orthostatic hypotension |
| Diuretics | Hypokalemia, hyperlipidemia, hyperglycemia, hyperuricemia |
| ARBs | Angioedema, rash, hyperkalemia |
| Hydralazine | Lupus-like syndrome |

Which three drugs are proven to reduce morbidity and mortality?

1. Beta-blockers
2. Thiazide diuretics
3. ACE inhibitors

## HYPERLIPIDEMIA

When should a patient with no family history be screened for hyperlipidemia?

Men aged 35; women aged 45

How often should a patient with previously normal lipids be rechecked for hyperlipidemia?

Every 5 years

What should the low-density lipoprotein (LDL) level be in a patient with no or one risk factor(s) for coronary artery disease (CAD)?

<160

What is the goal LDL for a patient with known CAD or CAD equivalents?

<70

What is the goal LDL for patient with no known CAD but with two or more risk factors?

<130

What are some examples of CAD equivalents?

Diabetes, peripheral artery disease, abdominal aortic aneurysm, more than a 20% 10-year risk of developing coronary artery disease

What is a protective factor in terms of hyperlipidemia?

High-density lipoprotein (HDL) >60

**What is the mechanism for each of the following lipid-lowering agents?**

| | |
|---|---|
| Statins | 3-hydroxy-3-methylglutaryl coenzyme A (HMG-CoA) reductase inhibitors; ↓ LDL ↑ HDL |
| Nicotinic acid | Decreases lipolysis and prevents cholesterol synthesis by the liver; ↓ LDL ↑ HDL |
| Fibrates | Reduces triglycerides in very low-density lipoprotein (VLDL) and chylomicrons; ↑ HDL ↓ triglycerides |
| Bile acid sequestrants | Bind bile acids in the gut; ↓ LDL |

**What should you be concerned about in a patient on a statin complaining of muscle pain?**

Rhabdomyolysis

**How can you test for this?**

Check creatine kinase (CK)

**What side effect of statins should you screen for?**

Elevation in alanine aminotransferase (ALT)

# CORONARY ARTERY DISEASE

**What is CAD?**

Atherosclerosis leading to angina or MI

**What are the risk factors for CAD?**

**Major**
 Family (hx) (MI before age 55 in a
  male or 65 in a female)
 Diabetes
 Smoking
 Hyperlipidemia
 Hypertension
 Age: male >45, female >55
**Minor**
 Obesity
 Male sex
 Postmenopausal female
 Elevated plasma homocysteine

| | |
|---|---|
| What lifelong treatment has been shown to decrease mortality in a patient with CAD? | Aspirin, beta-blocker, statin, ACE inhibitor |
| What is stable angina? | Substernal chest pain (may radiate as well to arms, jaw, and so forth) due to ischemia that occurs both predictably and reproducibly at a certain level of exertion and relieved with rest/nitrates |
| What are some classic electrocardio-graphic (EKG) findings in a patient with angina? | ST depression or T-wave inversion |
| What is the treatment for acute angina? | Sublingual nitroglycerin up to three doses |
| What is the long-term treatment for angina? | Nitrates, aspirin, beta-blocker, statin, smoking cessation |
| What is unstable angina? | Angina occurring more frequently, unrelieved by nitroglycerin, or occurs at rest |
| How do you evaluate a patient with unstable angina? | EKG, cardiac enzymes, and, once stable, a cardiac stress test to risk stratify; angiography may be necessary |
| How should a patient with unstable angina be treated? | Hospitalization and treatment with nitroglycerin, aspirin, beta-blocker, ACE inhibitor, statin, heparin drip or Lovenox while on a cardiac monitor |
| When is a coronary artery bypass graft (CABG) indicated? | Failure of medical treatment with severe three-vessel disease; multiple vessel disease in a diabetic patient; or >50% stenosis of the left main artery; proximal significant left anterior descending (LAD) coronary artery stenosis with left ventricular (LV) dysfunction |
| What is Prinzmetal angina? | Angina due to coronary vasospasm that is usually nonexertional but can be exertional. Angiography is normal in these patients. |
| What is an MI? | Myocardial necrosis caused by ischemia |

What are the classic symptoms of an MI?

Crushing, substernal chest pain described as chest tightness or pressure. It can radiate to the left arm, neck, or jaw and can be associated with concomitant diaphoresis, shortness of breath, nausea, and vomiting.

What patients can present with nonclassic symptoms?

Diabetics and the elderly

What are the classic EKG changes associated with an MI?

ST elevation (Fig 2-1A) or depression, new left bundle branch block (LBBB), T-wave changes (Fig 2-1B)

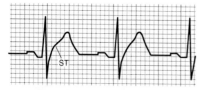

Figure 2-1A

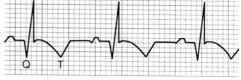

Figure 2-1B

What are defining factors for an MI?

Two of the following three being true:
1. New left bundle branch block
2. Chest pain >20 minutes
3. Elevated cardiac markers

What are the three different cardiac enzymes tested in a patient with chest pain?

Troponin, creatine kinase (CPK), and CK-MB (creatine kinase-MB)

How do the three cardiac enzymes differ in terms of elapsed time since an MI?

See Table 2-1.

**Table 2-1** Cardiac Enzyme Elevation in an Acute Myocardial Infarction

| Cardiac Enzyme | Troponin | CPK | CK-MB |
|---|---|---|---|
| Rises | 2-6 hours after injury | 4-6 hours | Within 3-4 hours |
| Peaks | 12-16 hours | 24 hours | Varies |
| Stays elevated for | 5-10 days | 2-3 days | 1-2 days |

| | |
|---|---|
| How often should the cardiac enzymes be done? | Repeat every 6-8 hours for a 24-hour period. |
| What is the mnemonic for emergent treatment of an MI? | Be MONA:<br><br>Beta-blocker<br>Morphine<br>Oxygen<br>Nitroglycerin<br>Aspirin |
| When is thrombolysis indicated? | In an ST-elevation MI, within 12 hours of onset of chest pain |
| What are contraindications to thrombolytics? | Previous cerebral hemorrhage, known cerebral aneurysm or arteriovenous malformation (AVM), known intracranial neoplasm, ischemic stroke in the last 3 months, aortic dissection, active bleeding, significant closed head or facial trauma |
| What is a contraindication to the use of streptokinase specifically? | Cannot be used more than once in a 6-month period because of its immunogenicity |
| What are some possible post-MI complications? | New arrhythmias; Dressler syndrome; papillary muscle rupture; thromboembolism; CHF, ventricular septal defect (VSD), myocardial rupture |
| What is Dressler syndrome? | An autoimmune process with the features of fever; pericarditis; elevated erythrocyte sedimentation rate (ESR) that occurs 2-4 weeks after an MI |
| What is the treatment of Dressler syndrome? | Nonsteroidal anti-inflammatory drugs (NSAIDs) and aspirin |
| What physical examination finding is indicative of a papillary muscle rupture? | New mitral regurgitation |

## ARRHYTHMIAS

Define each of the following types of heart block:

See Fig 2-2A-D.

    First-degree

PR interval is >0.2 seconds but all atrial impulses are conducted.

    Second-degree Mobitz type I

Also known as Wenckebach; PR intervals progressively increase until a beat is dropped

    Second-degree Mobitz type II

PR intervals are fixed with intermittently dropped QRS complexes.

    Third-degree

Also known as complete heart block; dissociation between atrial and ventricular activity; no relationship between P waves and QRS intervals

What is the treatment for each of the following types of heart block?

    1. First-degree

1. No treatment required

    2. Second-degree Mobitz type I

2. If caused by a drug, stop offending drug; may need a pacemaker if bradycardic

    3. Second-degree Mobitz type II

3. Pacemaker, because it can progress to third-degree block

    4. Third-degree

4. Pacemaker

Name some medications that can lead to second-degree heart block?

Digoxin, beta-blockers, calcium channel blockers

What is the most common chronic arrhythmia?

Atrial fibrillation

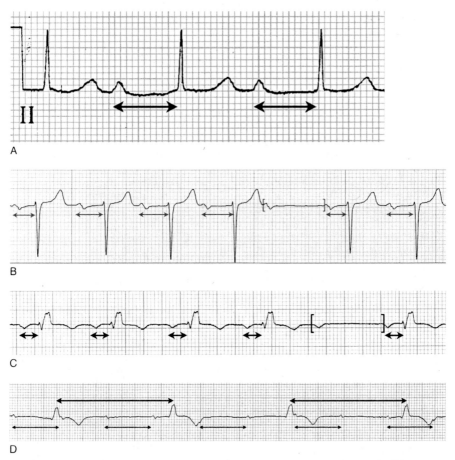

**Figure 2-2A-D**   **(A)** The PR interval is fixed (double arrows) and is >0.2 seconds, or five small blocks. **(B)** The PR interval gradually increases (double arrows) until a P wave is not followed by a QRS and a beat is "dropped" (brackets). The process then recurs. P waves occur at regular intervals, though they may be hidden by T waves. **(C)** The PR interval is constant (double arrows) until the dropped beat (brackets). **(D)** The P-P interval is uniform (lower double arrows) and the R-R interval is uniform (upper double arrows), but the P waves and QRS complexes are disassociated. *(Reproduced, with permission, from Knoop KJ, Stack LB, Storrow AB, et al. Atlas of Emergency Medicine. 3rd ed. New York: McGraw-Hill; 2010:747-750.)*

**What is atrial fibrillation?**

Irregularly irregular rhythm caused by disorganized electric activity of the atrium (Fig 2-3)

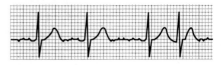

**Figure 2-3**

**What is the mnemonic for some etiologies of atrial fibrillation?**

PIRATES:

Pulmonary disease

Ischemia

Rheumatic heart disease

Anemia/Atrial myxoma

Thyroid

Ethanol

Surgery, Sepsis

**What is the most common underlying cause of atrial fibrillation?**

Chronic hypertension

**What are some symptoms that patients with atrial fibrillation complain of?**

Fatigue, light-headedness, palpitations

**What is the major complication of atrial fibrillation if left untreated?**

Embolization which often can lead to stroke

**What are the treatments of atrial fibrillation?**

**Rate control** with beta-blocker, calcium channel blocker (diltiazem), digoxin

**Antiarrhythmic agents** (if failure to rate control or symptomatic despite rate control)

**Anticoagulation** with Coumadin

In an unstable patient, synchronized cardioversion

**What is atrial flutter?**

Macroreentrant arrhythmia; atrial rates are typically between approximately 240 and 400 beats/min

**What is the classic EKG pattern described in atrial flutter?**

"Saw tooth" (Fig 2-4)

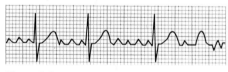

Figure 2-4

| | |
|---|---|
| **What is multifocal atrial tachycardia (MAT)?** | Irregularly irregular rhythm caused by at least three sites of competing atrial activity |
| **What is the classic EKG finding in MAT?** | At least three different P-wave morphologies in the same lead (Fig. 2-5) |

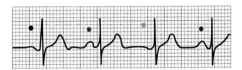

**Figure 2-5**

| | |
|---|---|
| **What medical condition is associated with MAT?** | COPD |
| **What is the treatment for MAT?** | Treat the underlying cause. |
| **What is a premature ventricular contraction (PVC)?** | Ectopic beats of ventricular origin |
| **What is the typical EKG finding in PVCs?** | Wide QRS with no P wave |
| **What is ventricular tachycardia (VT)?** | More than three consecutive PVCs; sustained VT must last >30 seconds (Fig 2-6) |

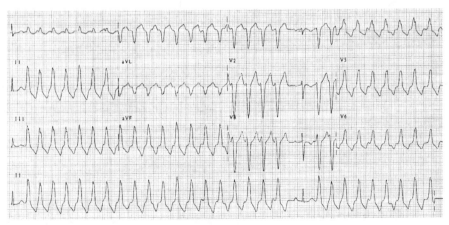

**Figure 2-6**    Ventricular tachycardia with capture beat. *(Reproduced, with permission, from Knoop KJ, Stack LB, Storrow AB, et al. Atlas of Emergency Medicine. 3rd ed. New York: McGraw-Hill; 2010:765. Photo contributor: James V. Ritchie, MD.)*

| | |
|---|---|
| **What is the possible complication of VT?** | Ventricular fibrillation or cardiac arrest/ hemodynamic collapse |
| **What is the treatment for VT?** | If the patient is asymptomatic and not hypotensive, treat with lidocaine or amiodarone; if the patient is hypotensive or pulseless, treatment is defibrillation. |
| **What is ventricular fibrillation?** | Disorganized electric activity of the ventricle (Fig 2-7) |

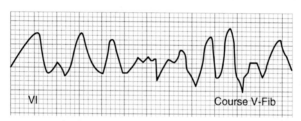

**Figure 2-7**

| | |
|---|---|
| **What is the treatment for ventricular fibrillation?** | Emergent cardioversion |
| **What is torsades de pointes?** | Prolonged VT with rotation around the axis in a patient with a prolonged QT interval at baseline |
| **What are the underlying causes of torsades de pointes?** | Quinine, procainamide, intracranial bleed, tricyclics, phenothiazines, electrolyte abnormalities such as hypomagnesemia, hypokalemia, hypocalcemia |
| **What are the classic EKG findings in Wolff-Parkinson-White (WPW) syndrome?** | "Delta" waves and short PR interval (Fig 2-8) |

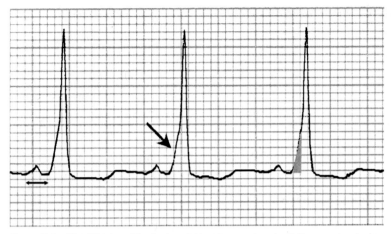

**Figure 2-8**   The PR interval is shortened (double arrow) and a delta wave (upsloping initial QRS segment) is seen (arrow, shaded area). *(Reproduced, with permission, from Knoop KJ, Stack LB, Storrow AB, et al. Atlas of Emergency Medicine. 3rd ed. New York: McGraw-Hill; 2010:775.)*

| | |
|---|---|
| **What medications are contraindicated in WPW?** | ABCD:<br>Adenosine<br>Beta-blocker<br>Calcium channel blocker<br>Digoxin |
| **What is the primary medical treatment for WPW?** | Procainamide |
| **What would be the first-line treatment in a WPW patient with hypotension, tachycardia, and evidence of hypoperfusion?** | Synchronized cardioversion because this patient is unstable |
| **How does digoxin toxicity present?** | Supraventricular tachycardia (SVT) with atrioventricular (AV) block and yellow vision |

## CONGESTIVE HEART FAILURE

| | |
|---|---|
| **What is the definition of CHF?** | Inability of the heart to pump enough blood to meet systemic demands. Left-sided heart failure (LHF) leads to pulmonary vascular congestion while right-sided heart failure (RHF) causes systemic venous congestion. |

| | |
|---|---|
| What are the underlying causes of CHF? | Myocardial ischemia, anemia, pulmonary embolism, endocarditis, cardiomyopathy, hypertension, pericarditis, cardiac dysrhythmias, thyrotoxicosis, diabetes, rheumatic heart disease, CAD |
| What is the most common cause of RHF? | Left heart failure |
| What are the symptoms of RHF? | Hepatomegaly, jugular venous distension (JVD), ascites |
| What are the symptoms of LHF? | Orthopnea, $S_3$ gallop, paroxysmal nocturnal dyspnea, cough, diaphoresis, rales |
| What is classically seen on a chest x-ray (CXR) in a patient with CHF? | Pulmonary vascular congestion, enlarged heart, curly B lines |
| What are the treatments for CHF? | ACE inhibitor, diuretics, digoxin, calcium channel blocker, sodium-restricted diet, beta-blockers (but not in acute CHF) |
| What is second-line treatment for CHF? | Isosorbide and hydralazine if the patient can't tolerate an ACE inhibitor |
| | ACE inhibitors, nitroprusside |
| What medications decrease afterload? | Diuretics, morphine, nitroglycerine |
| What medications decrease preload? | |
| Which medications have been shown to decrease mortality in CHF? | ACE inhibitor, beta-blocker, spironolactone (in class 3 and 4 heart failure) |
| What is initially used to treat acute pulmonary edema? | Remember the mnemonic MOrFiN |
| | Morphine |
| | Oxygen |
| | r |
| | Furosemide |
| | i |
| | Nitrates |

Name the drug(s) used in CHF that:

| | |
|---|---|
| Reduces afterload | ACE inhibitor |
| Is used for acute fluid retention | Loop diuretics |
| Are positive inotropes | Dobutamine, Dopamine, Digitalis |

## VALVULAR HEART DISEASES

| | |
|---|---|
| What does the $S_1$ sound represent in a heart beat? | Closure of mitral and tricuspid valves |
| What does the $S_2$ sound represent in a heart beat? | Closure of the aortic and pulmonic valves |
| What is the most common valvular heart disease found in young women? | Mitral valve prolapse |
| What is the underlying etiology of mitral valve prolapse? | Idiopathic; genetic transfer via autosomal dominant gene; ischemic heart disease; Marfan; myxomatous degeneration of the mitral valve |
| What is the pathognomonic murmur heard in a mitral valve prolapsed? | Late systolic murmur and a mid-systolic click |
| Where is the murmur most audible? | Apex |
| What is the treatment for mitral valve prolapse? | No treatment is necessary. |
| What are the underlying etiologies of mitral stenosis? | Most commonly due to **rheumatic heart disease** |
| In what sex does mitral stenosis predominate? | Females |
| What are the signs and symptoms of mitral stenosis? | Dyspnea, orthopnea, cough, rales, hoarse voice, atrial fibrillation, hemoptysis |
| What is the underlying cause leading to the symptoms found in mitral stenosis? | Flow is decreased behind the mitral valve leading to left atrial enlargement and eventually heart failure. |
| Name the valvular heart diseases that cause a systolic ejection murmur. | Pulmonary stenosis, aortic stenosis |

Name the valvular heart diseases that cause a pansystolic murmur.

Mitral regurgitation, tricuspid regurgitation

Name the valvular heart diseases that cause a diastolic murmur.

Aortic regurgitation

Name the valvular heart disease associated with each of the following:

Systolic crescendo-decrescendo murmur at the second right intercostal space, which radiates to carotids

Aortic stenosis

Mid-diastolic murmur with an opening snap and rumble best heard at the left sternal border

Mitral stenosis

Holosystolic murmur that radiates to the axilla

Mitral regurgitation

High-pitched decrescendo diastolic murmur, louder if leading forward

Aortic regurgitation

Diastolic murmur louder with inspiration

Tricuspid stenosis

Holosystolic murmur at the left lower sternal border

Tricuspid regurgitation

Late-systolic murmur with mid-systolic click

Mitral valve prolapse

What is a mnemonic to remember diastolic murmurs?

AR/MS piTS (Aortic Regurgitation/ Mitral Stenosis, Tricuspid Regurgitation)

What is a mnemonic to remember holosystolic murmurs?

MoR/TaR (Mitral Regurgitation/ Tricuspid Regurgitation)

# CARDIOMYOPATHY

What are the three categories of cardiomyopathy?

Remember the mnemonic HaRD

Hypertrophic

a

Restrictive

Dilated

| | |
|---|---|
| What is the mnemonic for some etiologies of a dilated cardiomyopathy? | **ABCD I**<br>Alcohol abuse<br>Beriberi<br>Cocaine, Chagas disease, Coxsackie B<br>Doxorubicin<br>Idiopathic, Ischemic, Infectious |

Name the type of cardiomyopathy associated with each of the following descriptions:

| | |
|---|---|
| Symptoms of CHF, $S_3$ heart sound, enlarged balloon–like heart, atrial fibrillation, mitral regurgitation, systolic dysfunction | Dilated |
| 50% of cases are genetically inherited via an autosomal dominant trait | Hypertrophic |
| Diastolic dysfunction as a result of ventricular enlargement and thickened septum, and systolic dysfunction as a result of LV outflow obstruction | Hypertrophic |
| Caused by radiation-induced fibrosis, endomyocardial fibrosis, amyloidosis, sarcoidosis, glycogen storage diseases | Restrictive |
| Syncope with exertion | Hypertrophic |
| Most common cause of sudden death in young adults | Hypertrophic |
| Mitral regurgitation, $S_4$ heart sound, systolic ejection murmur, large boot–shaped heart | Hypertrophic |
| Systolic dysfunction and left ventricular dilation are necessary to make the diagnosis | Dilated |
| Similar to constrictive pericarditis | Restrictive |
| Treatment includes cessation of all alcohol use | Dilated |
| Symptoms relieved with beta-blockers or calcium channel blockers | Hypertrophic |
| Treated with ACE inhibitor, beta-blocker, CHF-directed therapies, diuretics | Dilated |

# ENDOCARDITIS

**What is endocarditis?**

Heart valve inflammation usually due to an infective cause

**Name the most common causes of the following types of endocarditis:**

**Acute**

Most commonly, *Staphylococcus aureus* (IVDA [intravenous drug abuse]); others: *Streptococcus pneumoniae, Neisseria gonorrhoeae*

**Subacute**

Most commonly, *Streptococcus viridans* (dental work); others: *Enterococcus, Staphylococcus*

**Culture negative**

**HACEK:**

*Haemophilus influenza*

*Actinobacillus*

*Cardiobacterium*

*Eikenella*

*Kingella*

**Marantic**

Previous rheumatic fever or cancer metastasis

**What type of endocarditis is seen in systemic lupus erythematosus (SLE)?**

Libman-Sacks endocarditis (LSE) caused by autoantibodies damaging heart valves

**How can this be distinguished on echocardiogram?**

Sterile fibrofibrinous vegetations that favor the left-sided heart valves. They tend to form on the ventricular surface of the mitral valve.

**What are the signs and symptoms of endocarditis?**

Fever, chills, **Janeway lesion, Roth spots, Osler nodes, splinter hemorrhages,** new murmur, conjunctival hemorrhages

**What are Janeway lesions?**

Dark hemorrhagic peripheral macules or painless nodules usually on palms and soles (Fig 2-9)

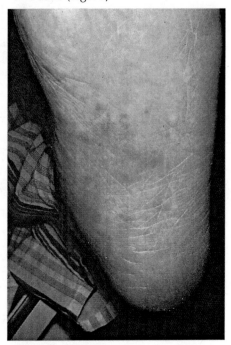

**Figure 2-9**   Janeway lesions. *(Reproduced, with permission, from Knoop KJ, Stack LB, Storrow AB, et al. Atlas of Emergency Medicine. 3rd ed. New York: McGraw-Hill; 2010:374. Photo contributor: Department of Dermatology, Wilford Hall USAF Medical Center and Brooke Army Medical Center, San Antonio, Texas.)*

**What are Roth spots?**

Retinal hemorrhages

**What are Osler nodes?**

Ouch! Painful nodules on fingers and toes (Fig 2-10)

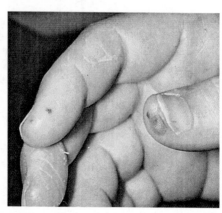

**Figure 2-10**    Osler nodes. *(Reproduced, with permission, from Knoop KJ, Stack LB, Storrow AB, et al.* Atlas of Emergency Medicine. *3rd ed. New York: McGraw-Hill; 2010:375. Photo contributor: Armed Forces Institute of Pathology, Bethesda, Maryland.)*

**What are splinter hemorrhages?**

Petechiae on fingernails (Fig 2-11)

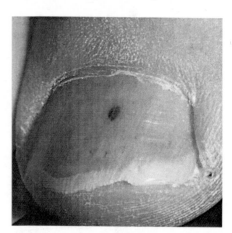

**Figure 2-11**    Splinter hemorrage. *(Reproduced, with permission, from Knoop KJ, Stack LB, Storrow AB, et al.* Atlas of Emergency Medicine. *3rd ed. New York: McGraw-Hill; 2010:375. Photo contributor: Armed Forces Institute of Pathology, Bethesda, Maryland.)*

**What is the most likely cause of right-sided endocarditis?**

IVDA

| | |
|---|---|
| What tests would you order to help diagnose endocarditis? | Three sets of blood cultures and an echocardiogram to look for vegetations |
| What valve is most commonly affected in endocarditis? | Mitral valve |
| What valve is most commonly affected in an IV drug user with infective endocarditis? | Tricuspid valve |
| What criteria are used to make the diagnosis of endocarditis? | Duke criteria |

What are the major criteria?

1. Two positive blood cultures demonstrating the same organism
2. Positive echocardiogram

What are the minor criteria?

1. Predisposing condition such as a valvular heart abnormality, hypertrophic cardiomyopathy, congenital heart disease
2. Documented temperature >38°C
3. Signs of embolic disease such as Janeway lesions, pulmonary emboli, cerebral emboli, hepatic or splenic emboli
4. Immunologic signs such as Roth spot
5. One positive blood culture

| | |
|---|---|
| Before an organism is isolated and antibiotics can be tailored, what antibiotics should be initiated in a patient suspected to have endocarditis? | Aminoglycoside and a beta-lactam |
| How long should a patient with endocarditis be treated with antibiotics? | 4-6 weeks |

Who should be treated with prophylactic antibiotics for endocarditis before dental procedures or gastrointestinal or genitourinary procedures?

Patients with any of the following:

History of endocarditis, prosthetic heart valves, unrepaired cyanotic heart disease, congenital cyanotic disease repaired within the last 6 months, or cardiac transplantation with subsequent valvulopathy

| | |
|---|---|
| What antibiotic is standard for prophylaxis prior to dental procedures? | Amoxicillin |

## RHEUMATIC FEVER

| | |
|---|---|
| **What infection causes rheumatic fever?** | Group A streptococcal pharyngitis |
| **Why does this infection cause rheumatic heart disease?** | The antistreptococcal antibodies react with cardiac antigen. |
| **What valve is most commonly affected in rheumatic heart disease?** | Mitral valve |
| **What serologic test could be used to confirm a prior streptococcal infection?** | A positive antistreptolysino (ASO) antibody titer |
| **What is the mnemonic for the five major criteria for rheumatic heart disease?** | **Jones** criteria:<br><br>**J**oints (migratory polyarthritis)<br>**C**arditis (endocarditis, pericarditis, myocarditis)<br>**N**odules (subcutaneous)<br>**E**rythema marginatum (serpiginous rash)<br>**S**ydenham chorea |
| **What are the minor criteria for rheumatic heart disease?** | PR-interval prolongation<br>Fever<br>Elevated ESR<br>Arthralgias |
| **How should streptococcal pharyngitis be treated to prevent rheumatic heart disease?** | Penicillin |

# PERICARDITIS

| | |
|---|---|
| What is pericarditis? | Inflammation of the pericardium |
| What are some causes of pericarditis? | Infectious: viral, bacterial, fungal<br><br>Autoimmune: rheumatoid arthritis, SLE, scleroderma<br><br>Drugs HIP: hydralazine, isoniazid, procainamide (these are the same drugs that can lead to SLE-like reaction); radiation therapy<br><br>Trauma<br><br>Post-MI<br><br>Metastatic cancer<br><br>Uremia |
| What is pericarditis that occurs 2-4 weeks post-MI called? | Dressler syndrome |
| What are the classic symptoms of pericarditis? | Pleuritic chest pain that is relieved with sitting up and leaning forward |
| What are the pathognomonic physical exam findings of pericarditis? | Pericardial **friction rub** on auscultation of the heart during expiration; **pulsus paradoxus** |

**What are the classic EKG findings associated with pericarditis?**

Diffuse ST elevations and PR depressions (usually in all or almost all leads) (Fig 2-12)

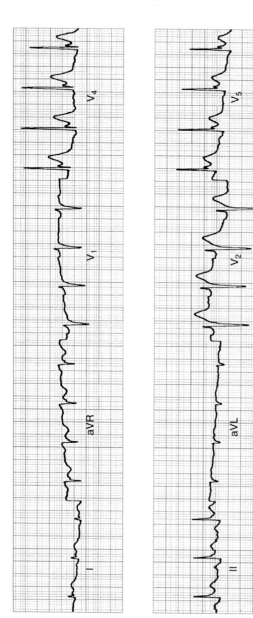
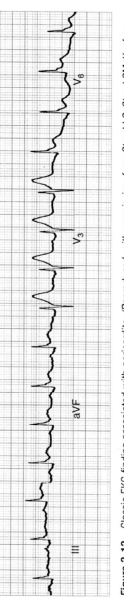

**Figure 2-12**    Classic EKG finding associated with pericardits. (Reproduced, with permission, from Stead LG, Stead SM, Kaufman MS, et al: First Aid for the Medicine Clerkship. 2nd ed. New York: McGraw-Hill; 2006:33.)

How can the diagnosis of pericarditis be confirmed? | Pericarditis is a clinical diagnosis, but an echocardiogram may show a pericardial effusion.

How is pericarditis treated? | The underlying cause should be addressed. NSAIDs to decrease inflammation; antibiotics for bacterial causes; steroids for autoimmune etiology; pericardiocentesis would be necessary for a large pericardial effusion

# MYOCARDITIS

What is myocarditis? | Inflammation of the heart muscle

What is the most common viral cause of myocarditis? | Enterovirus infection (eg, Coxsackie B)

What are the causes of myocarditis? | Viral: Coxsackie A and B, HIV, EBV (Epstein-Barr), HBV (hepatitis B), cytomegalovirus (CMV)

Bacterial: rheumatic fever, Lyme disease, meningococcus, mycoplasma

Parasitic: Chagas disease, toxoplasmosis, trichinella

Autoimmune: SLE, Kawasaki disease

Drugs

What are the signs and symptoms of myocarditis? | Precordial chest pain with signs of CHF

What does the EKG look like in a patient with myocarditis? | Nonspecific ST changes, dysrhythmias

How can a definitive diagnosis of myocarditis be made? | Myocardial biopsy

What is the treatment for myocarditis? | Treat CHF symptoms, dysrhythmias, and the underlying etiology. Steroids are contraindicated. In some cases, intravenous immunoglobulin (IVIG) is beneficial.

# CARDIAC TAMPONADE

What is cardiac tamponade?

Pericardial fluid accumulation that causes impaired cardiac filling and thus leads to decreased cardiac output

What is Beck's triad?

Symptoms seen in cardiac tamponade:
1. **Hypotension**
2. **Distant heart sounds**
3. **JVD**

What are some other classic symptoms of cardiac tamponade?

Dyspnea, tachycardia, pulsus paradoxus

What is pulsus paradoxus?

>10 mm Hg fall in blood pressure during inspiration

What is seen on EKG in a patient with pulsus paradoxus?

Electrical alternans—a beat-to-beat change in the height of the QRS complex

What study can help confirm the diagnosis of cardiac tamponade?

Echocardiogram will show a pericardial effusion.

What is the treatment for pericardial tamponade?

Pericardiocentesis vs pericardial window. IV fluids should also be given for volume expansion.

# ABDOMINAL AORTIC ANEURYSM

Who should be screened for an abdominal aortic aneurysm (AAA)?

Men older than 65 with a smoking history

What is the screening tool used?

Ultrasound

How should AAA be managed?

AAA <5 cm: blood pressure control, smoking cessation, and annual imaging

AAA >5 cm: elective surgical repair

What are the typical symptoms of a ruptured aneurysm?

Severe chest pain with radiation to the back between the scapula. Often described as a tearing pain.

| What is the treatment of a ruptured aneurysm? | Emergent surgery |
| What are the risk factors to the development of an AAA? | 1. Smoking (#1 risk factor)<br>2. Hyperlipidemia<br>3. Chronic hypertension |
| What is the classic description of a patient with an AAA on chest x-ray? | Widened mediastinum |

## CLINICAL VIGNETTES

A 54-year-old male with type II diabetes comes in for a routine physical. The vitals show a BP of 138/69. The patient currently takes aspirin, Zocor, and metformin. What type of drug would you add to this regimen?

ACE inhibitor

A 65-year-old male with a history of long-standing hypertension, presents with sensation of lightheadedness, shortness of breath, and palpitations. An EKG shows an irregularly, irregular rhythm. The heart rate is 110. The patient is started on a beta-blocker and the rate is controlled. You decide to start Coumadin. What is the goal INR?

INR between 2 and 3

A patient with a history of coronary artery disease presents to the emergency room complaining of chest pain. His medication list includes the following drugs: Prozac, lisinopril, atenolol, Zyrtec, nitroglycerin, aspirin, daily multivitamin. What class of medication would you suggest him to add to this regimen?

Statin

An obese 48-year-old male presents complaining of palpitations and light-headedness. An EKG demonstrates an irregularly irregular rhythm at 120 beats/min. What is the most likely underlying cause of this patient's problem?

The patient has atrial fibrillation and most likely caused by hypertension.

A 36-year-old male with no past medical history complains of several days of chest pain. The chest pain is exacerbated with inspiration and relieved with sitting up. He recently had a viral illness with fever. His physical examination is unremarkable. His EKG shows diffuse ST-segment elevations. What is the most likely diagnosis for this patient's symptoms and what is the first-line treatment?

Pericarditis and NSAIDs

# CHAPTER 3

# Pulmonology

## LUNG VOLUMES

What is the definition of each of the following? (Fig 3-1)

See Figure 3-1

Tidal volume (TV)

The air that is inhaled and exhaled during a normal respiration

Residual volume (RV)

Air that remains in the lungs after a maximal respiration

Inspiratory reserve volume (IRV)

Air in excess of TV that enters the lungs at maximal inspiration

Expiratory reserve volume (ERV)

Air that can be expired from the lungs after a normal expiration

Functional residual capacity (FRC)

RV + ERV

Inspiratory capacity (IC)

TV + IRV

Total lung capacity (TLC)

TV + IRV + RV + ERV

Vital capacity

TLC – RV

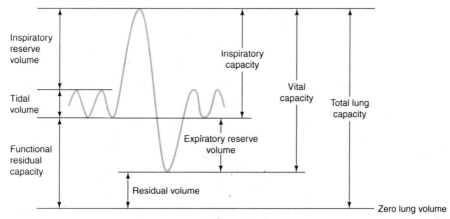

**Figure 3-1** Lung volumes as represented by spirogram tracing. *(This figure was published in Lumb AB. Nunn's Applied Respiratory Physiology, 5th ed. Butterworth-Heinemann. Copyright Elsevier 2000.)*

# HYPOXIA

| | |
|---|---|
| **What is the mnemonic for the mechanisms of hypoxia?** | **CIRCULAR:**<br>Circulatory<br>Increased oxygen requirement<br>Respiratory<br>Carbon monoxide poisoning<br>Underutilization<br>Low fraction of inspired oxygen ($F_{IO_2}$)<br>Anemia<br>Right-to-left shunt |
| **What are the important respiratory causes of hypoxia?** | Hypoventilation due to a decreased respiratory rate, decreased vital capacity, or ventilation/perfusion ratio (V/Q) mismatch |
| **How can respiratory hypoxia be improved?** | Supplemental oxygen and by treating the underlying cause |
| **What is a common underlying cause of decreased respiratory rate?** | Drugs: opiates |
| **What are common underlying causes of increased respiratory rate?** | Infection<br>Trauma |
| **What are some reasons for decreased vital capacity?** | Underlying lung disease, deformities of the chest wall such as in severe scoliosis, muscle weakness |
| **When is low $F_{IO_2}$ mostly a problem?** | High altitudes or closed spaces with no fresh air or fire |
| **How does diffusion impairment cause hypoxia?** | With circulatory impairment such as in heart failure or anemia, there is poor perfusion and, therefore, decreased blood transit time in the lungs causing decreased diffusion. Other reasons for diffusion impairment would be due to underlying lung pathology causing an increased diffusion pathway. |

| | | |
|---|---|---|
| Give an example of hypoxia caused by underutilization. | When there is impairment of cytochrome due to toxins/poisons, such as with cyanide | |
| What are the examples of increased requirement for oxygen? | Exercise, hyperthyroidism, infection | |
| What are some examples of causes of V/Q mismatch? | Pulmonary embolism, underlying lung disease such as in lung cancer or chronic obstructive pulmonary disease (COPD), bronchospasm, pneumonia, pulmonary edema | |
| Why is carbon monoxide poisoning a cause of tissue hypoxemia? | Carbon monoxide binds to hemoglobin and makes it unavailable for oxygen transport. | |
| What is the clinical sign of carbon monoxide poisoning? | Cherry red lips and nails | |
| What is an A-a gradient? | The difference in concentration between alveolar and arterial oxygen. It is a measure of gas exchange efficiency in the lung. The less the gradient the greater the oxygenation. | |

How do you expect the $P_{CO_2}$, and A-a gradient to be affected in each of the following causes of hypoxia?

1. Hypoventilation

2. Right-to-left shunt

3. Low $F_{IO_2}$

4. V/Q mismatch

See Table 3-1.

**Table 3-1** Hypoxia Etiology and Effects on $P_{CO_2}$ and A-a Gradient

| | Hypoventilation | R to L Shunt | Low $F_{IO_2}$ | V/Q Mismatch |
|---|---|---|---|---|
| $P_{CO_2}$ | ↑ | ↑ | normal | normal |
| A-a gradient | normal | ↑ | normal | ↑ |

| | |
|---|---|
| What are the signs and symptoms of hypoxia? | Dyspnea, tachypnea, tachycardia (increased perfusion), clubbing of nails, and cyanosis of extremities |

| | |
|---|---|
| What is the treatment for most types of hypoxia? | Increased $FiO_2$ via oxygen administration while identifying and treating the underlying cause |
| What type of hypoxemia does not improve with increased $FiO_2$? | A **right-to-left shunt** because there is no ventilation of the abnormal alveoli and, therefore, blood does not come in contact with oxygen |
| How is hypoxemia secondary to high altitude treated? | Oxygen administration can help but the body adjusts and self-corrects within several weeks. |

## OBSTRUCTIVE PULMONARY DISEASES

| | |
|---|---|
| What defines chronic obstructive pulmonary disease (COPD)? | As the name implies, it is defined by chronic obstruction to expiratory airflow such that the forced expiratory volume in 1 second/forced vital capacity ($FEV_1$/FVC) is decreased. |
| What are the two main forms of COPD? | Emphysema and chronic bronchitis |
| What is the male-to-female ratio of emphysema? | Male:female = 10:1. |
| What defines emphysema? | Chronic obstructive expiratory airflow with **dilation of air spaces** caused by destruction of alveolar walls |
| What is the most common cause of emphysema? | Smoking |
| What type of emphysema does smoking cause? | **Centrilobular,** meaning that it affects the bronchioles (Hint: The "S" sound is in both smoking and centrilobular) |
| What causes panacinar emphysema? | **Alpha-1-antitrypsin deficiency** |
| What is the function of alpha-1-antitrypsin in the lung? | It protects the elastin in the lungs from proteolytic enzymes. |
| What are the pathognomonic symptoms associated with emphysema? | **Pursed lip breathing** (with prolonged expiratory phase), **barrel chest, hyperventilation;** classically described as a "**pink puffer**," weight loss |

**What is seen on a chest x-ray (CXR) in a patient with emphysema?**

Hyperinflation and hyperlucency of the lungs with flattening of the diaphragms; parenchymal bullae and subpleural blebs may be present; alveolar wall destruction

**What do you expect to see in arterial blood gases (ABGs) in a person with early-stage emphysema?**

Low $P_{CO_2}$ and normal/low $P_{O_2}$

**What is the long-term treatment for emphysema?**

**Smoking cessation!** Home oxygen, bronchodilators, steroids; pneumococcal and flu vaccines should be offered

**What defines chronic bronchitis?**

Productive cough on most days during 3 or more consecutive months for 2 or more consecutive years

**What is the difference in symptomatology in chronic bronchitis vs emphysema?**

Chronic bronchitis includes a persistent productive cough as well as more hypoxia than seen in emphysema, and patients are usually overweight.

**What is the pathognomonic description of a person with chronic bronchitis?**

"Blue bloater" because of $CO_2$ retention and hypoxia

**What do you expect to see in an ABG in a person with chronic bronchitis?**

High $P_{CO_2}$ and low $P_{O_2}$, compensated respiratory acidosis

**What are the potential complications associated with chronic bronchitis?**

Right heart failure (cor pulmonale), polycythemia, pneumonia, hepatomegaly

**What is the treatment for chronic bronchitis?**

Treatments are the same as that for emphysema and include smoking cessation, oxygen therapy, bronchodilators, and steroids, and, also, some treatment with antibiotics in exacerbations.

**What are the only treatments proven to extend life in COPD?**

Oxygen therapy and smoking cessation

**How is bronchiectasis defined?**

Pathologic dilatation of bronchioles caused by chronic inflammation and wall structure destruction

**What are some common etiologies of bronchiectasis?**

Cystic fibrosis, tuberculosis (TB), lung abscess, toxin inhalation

What is the underlying pathologic problem that results because of chronic dilatation of bronchioles?

The dilated bronchioles impede mucociliary clearance, favoring mucus pooling and colonization with bacteria and, therefore, further lung damage.

What are the most common pathogens that colonize the lung in an individual with bronchiectasis?

SHiPS:

Staphylococcus aureus

Haemophilus influenzae

i

Pseudomonas

Streptococcus pneumonia

How do you treat the organisms that most commonly infect the lung in bronchiectasis?

Third-generation cephalosporin

What are the signs and symptoms of bronchiectasis?

Halitosis, hemoptysis, chronic cough with sputum production

How can bronchiectasis be diagnosed?

High-resolution computed tomographic (CT) scan of the lungs will demonstrate bronchial dilatation as well as destruction

What is the pathognomonic sign seen on CT in a person with bronchiectasis?

**Tram track lung markings**

What is the treatment for bronchiectasis?

Antibiotics for infections, bronchodilators, oxygen, mucolytics, chest PT and, sometimes, lung transplant

How is asthma defined?

Reversible obstruction of airways secondary to airway inflammation, hypersecretion and, most importantly, bronchoconstriction that leads to a decreased peak flow and $FEV_1$

What is intrinsic asthma associated with?

Exercise-induced or upper respiratory infection (URI)–induced asthma

What is extrinsic asthma associated with?

Asthma caused by **eosinophilia** or increased immunoglobulin E (IgE) levels in response to Environmental antigens

When does asthma usually start and what is its usual course?

Asthma generally begins during childhood and usually resolves on its own by the early teenage years.

What is often the first symptom of asthma that a patient will often describe?

Nighttime cough (for some people this is the only symptom)

What are some of the major signs and symptoms of an acute asthma exacerbation?

Expiratory wheeze, shortness of breath, chest tightness, subcostal retractions, accessory muscle use, prolonged expiratory phase

What would spirometry show in an asthmatic?

Decreased $FEV_1$

How can it be confirmed that the wheezing is caused by asthma and not some other cause?

The wheezing resolves with bronchodilator therapy and the $FEV_1$ will increase by 10% or more.

What would an ABG show in an asthma attack?

Hypoxia and respiratory alkalosis

What is a sign of impending respiratory failure in a case of asthma?

ABG that shows normalizing $Pco_2$

What classic diagnosis should you think of if the complete blood count (CBC) of an asthmatic demonstrates eosinophilia?

Churg-Strauss syndrome

What are the different categories of asthma, what are their symptoms (Sx), and what is the treatment for each?

See Table 3-2.

What is the first-line treatment for an acute asthma exacerbation?

Oxygen, bronchodilators (includes beta-agonist and ipratropium [Atrovent]), and steroids

What is the second-line treatment for an acute asthma attack?

Subcutaneous epinephrine and $MgSO_4$

How can mild asthma refractory to aggressive beta-agonist therapy be treated?

Add an inhaled steroid.

When is systemic corticosteroid therapy indicated in asthma?

Daily or continuous asthma that is refractory to beta-agonist and inhaled steroids

What are some alternative therapies in asthma?

Leukotriene inhibitors, methylxanthines, immunomodulators, leukotriene receptor modifiers, and cromolyn sulfate. Also allergic desensitization in extrinsic asthma.

*RULE OF 2s*

**Table 3-2** Asthma Classification and Medical Management

| Asthma Type | Symptoms | Treatment |
|---|---|---|
| Mild intermittent | <2 × per week and nighttime Sx <2 × per month | Short-acting beta-agonist (albuterol) |
| Mild persistent | >2 × per week and nighttime >2 × per month | Short-acting beta-agonist and low-dose steroid inhaler |
| Moderate persistent | Daily asthma with nighttime >1 × per week | Long-acting bronchodilator and medium-dose steroid as well as short-acting rescue as needed |
| Severe persistent | Continuous symptoms | Systemic steroids and long-acting bronchodilators |

# RESTRICTIVE LUNG DISEASE

What is the definition of a restrictive lung disease?

Unlike obstructive lung disease, the $FEV_1/FVC$ **is normal to high**; it is the **total lung capacity (TLC)** that decreases

What are some examples of restrictive lung diseases?

Interstitial lung diseases, spaceoccupying lesions such as tumors; pleural effusions; neuromuscular diseases such as severe scoliosis, spinal cord trauma, and multiple sclerosis

What are some examples of interstitial lung diseases?

Anything that causes chronic lung injury such as asbestosis, acute respiratory distress syndrome (ARDS), coal mine dust, silicosis, berylliosis, chronic lung injury because of chronic infections, radiation

What is the pathognomonic description of an interstitial lung disease?

"Honeycomb lung"

What is the most common cause of atelectasis?

A postoperative patient who is nonambulatory for a long period of time

What types of chemotherapy can cause a restrictive lung disease?

Busulfan and bleomycin

# PLEURAL EFFUSION

What is a pleural effusion?

Increased fluid in the pleural space

What are the two main types of pleural effusions?

1. Exudate
2. Transudate

What are some common causes of exudative pleural effusions?

Infection such as pneumonia, malignancy, collagen vascular disease

What are some common causes of transudative pleural effusions?

Congestive heart failure (CHF), cirrhosis, nephritic syndrome

What is the underlying cause of fluid buildup in an exudate?

Increased capillary permeability

What is the underlying cause of fluid buildup in a transudate?

1. Decreased oncotic pressure
2. Increased hydrostatic pressure

How can a pleural effusion be evaluated?

Thoracentesis with analysis of cell counts, cultures, chemistries, and cytology

How can a pleural effusion be treated?

Treating the underlying cause and thoracentesis can be both diagnostic and therapeutic.

What lab tests should be sent in order to evaluate the pleural fluid?

Fluid and serum protein, glucose, lactate dehydrogenase (LDH); fluid culture and Gram stain; fluid cytology and cell count with differential and, additionally, you can send fluid amylase, AFB, ANA, RF, pH

What defines an exudative effusion?

If any of the following is true, the fluid effusion is considered exudative.

Pleural protein/serum protein >0.5

Pleural LDH/serum LDH >0.6

Pleural LDH >200

What does it signify if the pleural fluid has >10,000 WBCs with polymorphonuclear neutrophils (PMNs)?

Most likely a parapneumonic effusion

| | |
|---|---|
| What is gross blood in the pleural fluid associated with? | Tumor or trauma |
| What can low glucose (glucose <60) in the pleural fluid be associated with? | Tumor, empyema, rheumatologic etiology, parapneumonic exudate |
| What are high amylase levels in pleural fluid associated with? | Pancreatitis but can also be malignancy, or esophageal rupture |
| What percentage of pleural effusions caused by malignancy will have a fluid cytology that has malignant cells? | Only 40% 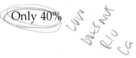 |
| How can exudative and transudative pleural effusions be differentiated? | See Table 3-3. |

**Table 3-3** Exudative vs. Transudative Pleural Effusion

| Test | Exudate | Transudate |
|---|---|---|
| Pleural LDH/serum LDH | >0.6 | <0.6 |
| Pleural LDH | >200 | <200 |
| Pleural protein/serum protein | >0.5 | <0.5 |
| Gram stain | Bacteria present most likely secondary to pneumonia (PNA) | No bacteria |
| WBC | >1000 | <1000 |
| Glucose | <60 | >60 |
| Differential | Parapneumonic, malignancy, rheumatologic disease | CHF, pulmonary embolism (PE), cirrhosis, nephritic syndrome |

# COUGH

| | |
|---|---|
| What is the definition of an acute cough? | Cough that has lasted <3 weeks |
| What is the most common cause of an acute cough? | Postnasal drip (also very common are asthma and GERD) |

**What are the most common causes of postnasal drip?**

Sinusitis, allergic rhinitis, seasonal or environmental allergies, flu or cold

**What is the preferred method of treatment of postnasal drip caused by allergies?**

Antihistamine treatment and/or nasal corticosteroid

**What is the preferred method of treatment of postnasal drip caused by the cold?**

Antihistamine as well as a decongestant

**What is sinusitis?**

A bacterial or viral infection of the sinuses

**Which sinus is most commonly affected?**

The maxillary sinus

**What are the signs and symptoms of sinusitis?**

Fever, tenderness to percussion over the sinuses, increased pain with bending forward, purulent nasal discharge, halitosis, headache

**Define acute, subacute, and chronic sinusitis?**

Acute sinusitis lasts <3 weeks, subacute lasts between 21 and 60 days, and chronic sinusitis lasts >60 days.

**What most commonly causes acute sinusitis?**

Viruses

**What are the most common pathogens involved in acute bacterial sinusitis?**

*Streptococcus pneumoniae, H influenzae,* and *Moraxella catarrhalis*

**What is the treatment for acute sinusitis?**

Viral rhinosinusitis does not require antimicrobial treatment. Nasal corticosteroids and decongestants are helpful. Studies have shown that steroids lead to faster symptom resolution. Bacterial causes should be treated with amoxicillin, augmentin, or bactrim for 1-2 weeks.

**What are the potential complications secondary to chronic sinusitis?**

Meningitis, osteomyelitis, orbital cellulitis, cavernous sinus thrombosis, abscess

| | |
|---|---|
| What is the classic organism causing sinusitis in a diabetic? | *Aspergillus* causing mucormycosis |
| What is the definition of a chronic cough? | A cough lasting >3 weeks |
| What are the three most common causes of chronic cough? | 1. Postnasal drip ✓<br>2. Asthma<br>3. Gastroesophageal reflux disease (GERD) |
| What medication class can cause a chronic cough? | Angiotensin–converting enzyme (ACE) inhibitors |

# ACUTE RESPIRATORY DISTRESS SYNDROME

| | |
|---|---|
| What are the components of acute respiratory distress syndrome (ARDS)? | Refractory hypoxemia, decreased lung compliance, noncardiogenic pulmonary edema |
| What is the etiology of ARDS? | Endothelial injury secondary to aspiration, multiple transfusions, shock, sepsis, trauma |
| What are the criteria needed to diagnose ARDS? | 1. Acute onset of respiratory distress<br>2. $P_{AO_2}$: $F_{IO_2}$ ratio <200 mm Hg<br>3. Bilateral pulmonary infiltrates on CXR<br>4. Normal capillary wedge pressure |
| What is the treatment for ARDS? | Treat the underlying disease and give adequate oxygen via mechanical ventilation |
| What is the overall mortality in ARDS? | About 50% |

# PULMONARY EMBOLISM

| | |
|---|---|
| What is the most common etiology of a pulmonary embolism (PE)? | Dislodged deep vein thrombosis (DVT) |
| What are the risk factors for a DVT? | Virchow triad: stasis (usually due to immobilization), hypercoagulable state, endothelial injury |
| What are the risk factors for a PE? | Same risk factors as getting a DVT, as well as having a DVT, stroke, myocardial infarction (MI); recent surgery leading to immobilization |
| What are some examples of hypercoagulable states? | Malignancy; protein C or protein S deficiency; antithrombin III deficiency; factor V Leiden deficiency; hyperestrogen states such as pregnancy, oral contraceptive use, smoking |
| What is an important question to ask in the patient's history? | Ask if they have had any recent travel or other immobilization. Long trips cause people to be immobile for long periods of time and therefore have a greater risk for developing DVTs and therefore PEs. |
| What is the most common sign in a patient with a PE? | Sinus tachycardia |
| What are some of the common symptoms of PE? | Dyspnea, tachypnea, pleuritic chest pain, fever, unilaterally swollen and painful posterior lower extremity, cough, hemoptysis |
| What are the classic CXR findings in a PE? | Hampton hump—wedge-shaped infarct<br>Westmark sign—hyperlucency in the lung region supplied by the affected artery |

**What is the most common EKG finding in a PE patient?**

Sinus tachycardia

**What is the classic EKG finding in a PE patient?**

S1Q3T3—S wave in lead I, Q wave in lead III, and inverted T wave in lead III (Fig 3-2)

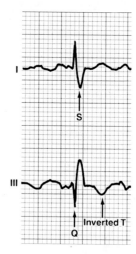

**Figure 3-2** Pulmonary embolism S1Q3T3 pattern. *(Reproduced with permission from Kaufman MS et al. First Aid for the Medicine Clerkship. New York: McGraw Hill; 2002:75; Figure 3-1)*

**What is the gold standard for diagnosis of PE?**

Pulmonary angiography

**What are some of the diagnostic techniques used to diagnose a PE?**

Spiral CT, V/Q scan, pulmonary angiography or MR angiography

**What blood test can be done to rule out PE if it is not positive?**

D-dimer

**What diagnostic test can be done to rule out a DVT?**

Duplex ultrasound

**What is the algorithm used to diagnose**     See Fig 3-3.
**a PE, when one is suspected?**

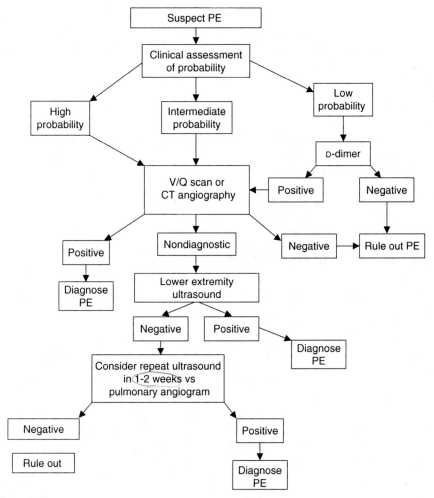

**Figure 3-3**

**What are the treatments for a PE?**     Heparin or Lovenox (low-molecular-
weight heparin) acutely, long-term
treatment with Coumadin or inferior
vena cava (IVC) filter, or tissue-type
plasminogen activator (tPA)
thrombolysis in massive PE

| | |
|---|---|
| What needs to be done if Coumadin is being started? | Heparin must be continued until Coumadin becomes therapeutic since Coumadin can cause a hypercoagulable state. |
| What is the therapeutic international normalized ratio (INR)? | INR of 2-3 |

# PNEUMOTHORAX

| | |
|---|---|
| A person with what body habitus is most likely to have a primary spontaneous pneumothorax? | Tall and thin male |
| What is the most likely etiology of a primary spontaneous pneumothorax? | Rupture of subpleural blebs |
| What are some risk factors for having a secondary spontaneous pneumothorax? | COPD, lung cancer, pneumonia, TB, HIV, cystic fibrosis, trauma |
| What are the signs and symptoms of a pneumothorax? | Sudden unilateral chest pain, dyspnea, and tachypnea |
| What is found on physical examination in a person with a pneumothorax? | Absent breath sounds on the side of the pneumothorax and hyperresonance to percussion |
| What is seen on CXR in a pneumothorax? | Absent lung markings on the side of the pneumothorax |
| What is the treatment of a spontaneous pneumothorax? | Oxygen is the mainstay of therapy, but if the pneumothorax is symptomatic, a tube thoracostomy may be indicated. Pleurodesis can be used to make the visceral and parietal pleura adhere to each other. |
| What is a tension pneumothorax? | A chest wall defect causes air to be trapped in the pleural space during expiration like a one-way valve (Fig 3-4). |

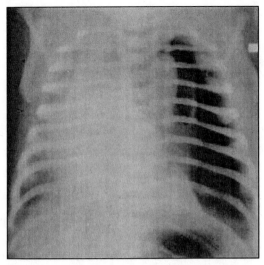

**Figure 3-4** Tension pneumothorax. *(Reproduced, with permission, from William Herring, MD, FACR; Radiology Residency Program Director at Albert Einstein Medical Center in Philadelphia, PA;* http://www.learningradiology.com*)*

| | |
|---|---|
| How is a tension pneumothorax treated? | This is a medical emergency. Treatment includes immediate needle decompression and chest tube placement thereafter. |

## HEMOPTYSIS

| | |
|---|---|
| What are the two most common causes of hemoptysis in the United States? | 1. Bronchitis<br>2. Bronchogenic carcinoma |
| What are the two most common causes of hemoptysis worldwide? | 1. Tuberculosis<br>2. Bronchiectasis |
| What are some other causes of hemoptysis? | Pneumonia, Wegener granulomatosis, Goodpasture syndrome, mycetoma, pneumonitis, arteriovenous (AV) malformation, pulmonary embolism, airway trauma, foreign body, metastatic lung tumor, bronchial carcinoid |
| What are the treatments for hemoptysis? | Have the patient lie down with the bleeding side down to protect the airway, oxygen as needed and in severe cases, bronchial artery embolization or intubation of the good lung |

## LUNG CANCER

| | |
|---|---|
| What is the most common cause of cancer death in the United States? | Lung cancer |
| What is the most likely causative factor of lung cancer? | Smoking |
| What are some other causes of lung cancer? | Second-hand smoke, exposure to asbestos, nickel, arsenic, radon gas |
| What are the two main categories of lung cancer? | Small cell and nonsmall cell |
| What are the different types of lung tumors that are nonsmall cell lung cancers? | Large cell, adenocarcinoma, squamous cell, bronchoalveolar cell |

Name the type of lung cancer associated with the following:

| | |
|---|---|
| Central location | Small cell, squamous cell |
| Poor response to chemotherapy | Nonsmall cell |
| Treated with surgery | Nonsmall cell |
| Poorer prognosis | Small cell |
| Sensitive to chemotherapy | Small cell |
| Peripheral location | Nonsmall cell |
| Linked to smoking | Small cell and squamous cell |
| Not linked to smoking | Bronchoalveolar cancer, a type of adenocarcinoma |
| Secretes parathyroid hormone-related peptide | Squamous cell |
| Associated with hypercalcemia | Squamous cell |
| Metastatic at diagnosis | Small cell |
| Secretes serotonin | Carcinoid tumor |
| Eaton-Lambert syndrome | Small cell |
| SIADH (syndrome of inappropriate antidiuretic hormone) | Small cell |
| Cushing syndrome | Small cell associated with adrenocorticotropic hormone (ACTH) secretion |
| Asbestos exposure | Mesothelioma |

| | |
|---|---|
| What are some signs and symptoms of lung cancer? | Chronic cough, hemoptysis, weight loss, night sweats, pneumonia (postobstructive), hoarseness, paraneoplastic syndrome |
| How is lung cancer diagnosed? | Usually a nodule or mass is seen on CXR or CT of the chest and is diagnosed with a biopsy usually done via bronchoscopy or CT-guided fine-needle aspiration |
| What are some of the signs and symptoms of a carcinoid tumor? | Symptoms of carcinoid syndrome due to serotonin secretion, which include flushing, asthmatic wheeze, diarrhea |
| What is the diagnostic test for a carcinoid tumor? | Test for elevated urine 5-hydroxyindoleacetic acid (5-HIAA), a serotonin metabolite |
| How is carcinoid syndrome treated? | Serotonin antagonist |
| What is a Pancoast tumor? | Superior sulcus tumor |
| What paraneoplastic syndromes are associated with a Pancoast tumor? | Horner syndrome, superior vena cava syndrome |
| What is Pancoast syndrome? | Shoulder and arm pain secondary to the tumor compressing the thoracic inlet with compression of the brachial plexus and cervical sympathetic nerves |

Name the paraneoplastic syndrome associated with signs and symptoms described below:

| | |
|---|---|
| Ptosis, myosis, anhydrosis | Horner syndrome |
| Facial and upper extremity swelling | Superior vena cava syndrome |
| Hyponatremia secondary to ectopic release of antidiuretic hormone (ADH) | SIADH |
| Low acetylcholine release leading to myasthenia gravis type symptoms | Eaton-Lambert syndrome |

Symptoms improve throughout day!

## PNEUMONIA

What are some common signs and symptoms of pneumonia (PNA)?

Cough with purulent sputum, fever, chills, pleuritic chest pain

What are some common physical examination findings in a patient with pneumonia?

Decreased breathing sounds, crackles, egophony, dullness to percussion, tactile fremitus on the side of the pneumonia, fever

What studies should be ordered if a PNA is suspected?

CXR, CBC, sputum culture and Gram stain, blood culture (in hospitalized patient)

What do you see on a CXR in a patient with pneumonia?

Lobar consolidation (Fig 3-5)

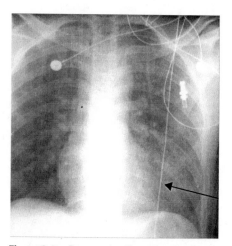

**Figure 3-5**    Pneumonia. *(Reproduced, with permission, from William Herring, MD, FACR; Radiology Residency Program Director at Albert Einstein Medical Center in Philadelphia, PA; http://www. learningradiology.com)*

| | |
|---|---|
| What would the CBC show? | Leukocytosis with a left shift ↗N⁷⁶ |
| Name the most common organism causing pneumonia in each of the following cases: | |
| Community-acquired pneumonia | *S pneumonia* |
| Typical community-acquired pneumonia | *S pneumoniae* and *H influenza* |
| Atypical community-acquired pneumonia | *Chlamydia*, *Legionella*, *Mycoplasma* — WALKING |
| Hospital-acquired pneumonia | *Pseudomonas*, *S aureus*, enteric gram-negative rods |
| Pneumonia in a patient with cystic fibrosis that easily develops resistance | *Pseudomonas* |
| Pneumonia after the flu | *S aureus* |
| Atypical pneumonia in the young patient, "walking pneumonia" | *Mycoplasma* |
| Right upper lobe pneumonia in an alcoholic | *Klebsiella*, usually secondary to aspiration |
| Positive cold agglutinin test | *Mycoplasma* |
| Pneumonia in a butcher who sells rabbit meat | *Francisella tularensis* |
| Pneumonia in a person who likes to explore caves in the Ohio Valley | *Histoplasma* |
| Pneumonia in a person from southwestern United States | *Coccidioides immitis* |
| Pneumonia in a bird keeper | *Chlamydia psittaci* |
| Pneumonia that mimics TB, and is gram positive | *Nocardia* |
| Pneumonia in a person with a lot of air-conditioning exposure or aerosolized water | *Legionella* |
| Aspiration pneumonia in an alcoholic, a patient with dementia, or a person who became unconscious | Anaerobes |
| Pneumonia contracted from farm animals and called "Q fever" | *Coxiella burnetii* |

| | |
|---|---|
| Pneumonia with hyponatremia, LDH >700, diarrhea, mental status change | *Legionella* |
| Fungus ball | *Aspergillus* |
| Rust-colored sputum | *S pneumonia* |
| Currant jelly sputum | *Klebsiella* |
| Three pneumonias in AIDS patients with CD4 count <200 | *Pneumocystis carinii, Histoplasma, Cryptococcus* |
| Pneumonia in AIDS patients with CD4 count < 50 | *Mycobacterium avium*, cytomegalovirus (CMV) |
| Bilateral infiltrates on CXR | *Mycoplasma, P carinii* pneumonia (also known as *Pneumocystis jiroveci*) |

**What is the treatment for each of the following cases of pneumonia?**

| | |
|---|---|
| Typical   Strep, HFLu | Third-generation cephalosporin plus macrolide or fluoroquinolone |
| Atypical   mycl, Chlamydia | Doxycycline, macrolide, quinolone |
| Anaerobic | Clindamycin, metronidazole |
| *P carinii* | Bactrim |

**What are the most common pathogens and treatments in each of the following cases?**

| | |
|---|---|
| Outpatient community-acquired pneumonia in a patient aged <60 | Organisms: *S pneumoniae, Mycoplasma, Chlamydia pneumoniae, H flu* (H influenzae) |
| | Treatment: erythromycin, tetracycline, or azithromycin to also cover *H flu* |
| Outpatient with age >60 and with comorbidities such as CHF, COPD, diabetes, alcoholic, cirrhosis | Organisms: *S pneumoniae, H flu,* aerobic gram-negative rods such as *Klebsiella, Escherichia coli, Enterobacter, S aureus, Legionella* |
| | Treatment: second-generation cephalosporin, amoxicillin, fluoroquinolone, erythromycin, or doxycycline for atypical pneumonia |
| Community-acquired pneumonia requiring hospitalization | Organisms: *S pneumoniae, H flu,* anaerobes, aerobic gram-negative rods, *Legionella, Chlamydia* |
| | Treatment: third-generation cephalosporin and azithromycin or doxycycline for atypical pneumonia |

| Community-acquired pneumonia requiring intensive care unit (ICU) admission | Organisms: *S pneumoniae, H flu, S aureus,* gram-negative bacilli, *Legionella, Pseudomonas* |
|---|---|
| | Treatment: third-generation cephalosporin and azithromycin or doxycycline for atypical pneumonia |
| Nosocomial pneumonia | Organisms: *Pseudomonas, S aureus, Legionella,* gram-negative rods |
| | Treatment: third-generation cephalosporin, aminoglycoside, or piperacillin tazobactam and vancomycin if methicillin-resistant *S aureus* (MRSA) suspected |

# TUBERCULOSIS

| How does TB spread? | Air droplet transmission |
|---|---|
| Who is at high risk for becoming infected with TB? | Immunocompromised, foreign-born, homeless, prisoner, low-income communities, intravenous (IV) drug users |
| What are the common signs and symptoms of TB? | **Productive cough, night sweats, weight loss, hemoptysis**, fever, chills, chest pain |
| How is latent TB detected? | Positive purified protein derivative (PPD) (tuberculin) skin test |
| What is considered a positive PPD? | >15 mm in any person |
| | >10 mm in immunocompromised, IV drug user, foreign-born, prisoner, nursing home resident, people who work in the medical field (that means you), underserved community |
| | >5 mm: HIV, abnormal CXR, close contact with someone who had TB |
| How is a positive PPD treated? | Isoniazid (INH) for 9 months with vitamin $B_6$ |
| What laboratory tests should be done when starting a patient on INH? | Liver function tests (LFTs) because of possibility of hepatotoxicity |

What part of the lung does primary TB usually affect?

Lower lobes

What is the radiographic finding of healed primary TB called?

"Ghon complex," which is a calcified nodule with calcified lymph nodes (Fig 3-6)

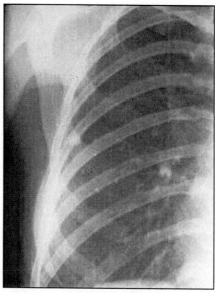

**Figure 3-6**   Tuberculosis. *(Reproduced, with permission, from William Herring, MD, FACR; Radiology Residency Program Director at Albert Einstein Medical Center in Philadelphia, PA; http://www.learningradiology.com)*

What is secondary TB?

Reactivation TB

Where is secondary TB usually found?

Lung apices

What is extrapulmonary TB?

TB that had disseminated to other organs

What is the most common extrapulmonary location for TB to spread?

Kidneys

What are other locations where extrapulmonary TB can be found?

Liver, central nervous system (CNS), vertebral bodies, psoas muscle, cervical lymph nodes, pericardium

What is TB of the vertebral bodies called?

Pott disease

What is cervical lymphadenopathy secondary to TB infection called?

Scrofula

How is active TB diagnosed?

Clinical symptoms, CXR, and sputum acid-fast stain and culture

What is seen on CXR in active TB?

Upper lobe infiltrates with scarring, cavitary lesions

What is the standard treatment for active TB?

Four-drug therapy initially for 2 months followed by 2-drug therapy (of INH and rifampin) for 4 months (remember the mnemonic **RIPE**):

Rifampin

**INH**

Pyrozinamide

Ethambutol

# CLINICAL VIGNETTES

A 63-year-old female with a history of ovarian cancer presents with severe shortness of breath and chest pain with inspiration. She has a low-grade fever, heart rate of 125, blood pressure of 138/60, respiratory rate of 25, and oxygen saturation of 88%. What test will confirm the diagnosis?

CT pulmonary angiogram or V/Q scan to check for a pulmonary embolism

A 30-year-old male with no significant past medical history presents to your office with fever, cough, and shortness of breath. On examination there are decreased breath sounds in the right lower lobe. His oxygen saturation is 92%. He has an elevated white count on CBC. What organism do you suspect?

*Mycoplasma*

A healthy American born 28-year-old male has started a new job at the bank that requires him to get a PPD. He denies exposure to tuberculosis and in a recent HIV test he had was negative. His PPD comes back at 16 mm. What is your next step?

Treat with INH and vitamin B$_6$ 9 months

A 60-year-old male with a 40 pack-year history of smoking presents with a cough. He states that the cough has been present for many months. It is a dry cough. He denies any chest pain or fever but does state that he often feels short of breath. A CBC comes back within normal limits. On examination he is a barrel-chested male with decreased breath sounds throughout and distant heart sounds. CXR only demonstrates flattened diaphragms. What is the most likely reason for this patient's cough?

Emphysema

A tall 20-year-old male complains of sudden left-sided chest pain with shortness of breath and tachypnea. The chest x-ray shows absent lung markings of the left side. What is the initial treatment for his condition?

Tension pneumothorax requires immediate needle decompression followed by chest tube placement

# CHAPTER 4

# Neurology

*TIA < RIND < STROKE*

## CEREBROVASCULAR ACCIDENTS

| | |
|---|---|
| What is a cerebrovascular accident (CVA)? | Sudden onset of neurologic deficit that is a result of cerebrovascular disease |
| What does TIA stand for? | Transient ischemic attack |
| What is a TIA? | A neurologic deficit that lasts **<24 hours and resolves completely** |
| What is a stroke? | Focal neurologic deficit that results from infarcted cerebral tissue |
| What does RIND stand for? | Reversible ischemic neurologic deficit |
| What is RIND? | Neurologic deficits that last >24 hours and <3 weeks |
| What are the two greatest risk factors for a stroke? | 1. Hypertension<br>2. Smoking |
| What are the two etiologies of a CVA? | Ischemic or hemorrhagic stroke |
| What are the two most common etiologies for ischemia? | 1. Thrombotic etiology which is secondary to atherosclerosis<br>2. Embolic etiology which is usually either cardiac in origin or from carotid arteries |
| What is the most common etiology of a CVA? | Ischemia |

Name the term associated with each of the following:

| | |
|---|---|
| Difficulty with expression of both written and spoken language as well as difficulty with comprehension | Aphasia |
| Difficulty with performing motor tasks | Apraxia (a patient with **apraxia** can't practice) |
| Difficulty with articulation | Dysarthria |
| CVA sequelae in which the patient speaks with fluency, however, without making sense, and comprehension is impaired and patient is unaware of the deficit | Wernicke aphasia (Wernicke is **wordy**) |
| CVA sequelae in which the patient has difficulty verbalizing what they want to express, comprehension is intact, and patient is aware of the deficit | Broca aphasia (Broca had **broken** language) |
| Infarct in the deep gray matter associated with hypertension and atherosclerosis | Lacunar infarct |
| Infarction that occurs in an area supplied by two major arteries and is usually a result of hypotension | Watershed infarct |
| Most common source of emboli that leads to a stroke | Carotid atheroma |
| Thalamus, internal capsule, and cerebral white matter deficit causing *flexion* of the upper extremities | Decorticate posturing |
| Upper brain stem deficit causing *extension* of the upper extremities | Decerebrate rigidity |

Describe the deficits caused by
occlusion of the following arteries:

| | |
|---|---|
| Middle cerebral artery (MCA) supplying the dominant hemisphere | Contralateral hemiparesis and hemisensory deficit, aphasia, homonymous hemianopsia |
| MCA supplying the nondominant hemisphere | Contralateral hemiparesis and hemisensory deficit, homonymous hemianopsia, confusion, apraxia, body neglect on contralateral side |
| Anterior cerebral artery (ACA) | Broca aphasia, contralateral weakness of lower extremity, incontinence |
| Posterior cerebral artery (PCA) | Homonymous hemianopsia with macular sparing, oculomotor nerve palsy, aphasia, and alexia if dominant hemisphere is affected |
| Posterior inferior cerebellar artery (PICA) | Vertigo, ataxia, contralateral pain and temperature disturbance, dysphagia, dysarthria, ipsilateral Horner syndrome (ptosis, miosis, anhidrosis) |
| Anterior inferior cerebellar artery | Deafness, tinnitus, ipsilateral facial weakness, gaze palsy |
| Ophthalmic artery | Amaurosis fugax (transient monocular blindness) |
| What is the first study to order if you suspect a stroke in a patient? | Computed tomography (CT) of head **without** contrast to rule out a bleed |
| What other studies can be done to further assess the patient? | Magnetic resonance imaging (MRI) to evaluate for subacute infarction; carotid Doppler ultrasound to rule out carotid artery stenosis; echocardiogram to rule out embolic sources |
| What is the treatment for a TIA? | Patient should be started on aspirin. |
| What medication should the patient be started on if they fail aspirin? | Plavix (clopidogrel) |
| What other antiplatelet therapies are available other than aspirin? | Plavix (clopidogrel), ticlopidine, Aggrenox |
| When would you consider a carotid endarterectomy? | If the patient had carotid artery stenosis >70% |
| What is the treatment for a patient who had a cardioembolic stroke? | Anticoagulation with heparin or Coumadin |

| | |
|---|---|
| What treatment improves outcome in a patient who present with an embolic stroke with symptoms beginning <3 hours ago? | Tissue plasminogen activator (tPA) |
| What is the major contraindication to tPA use? | Intracranial bleeding |
| How should hypertension be treated in a patient who acutely had a stroke? | Hypertension should not acutely be controlled tightly in order to allow for good cerebral perfusion. A 25% reduction in mean arterial pressure in the first 24 hours is acceptable. |
| Other than starting medications, what other long-term interventions should be taken in a patient with a history of stroke to prevent future infarctions? | Good diabetes control (improved HgA1c); control hypertension; smoking cessation; treat hyperlipidemia |

## SEIZURE DISORDERS

| | |
|---|---|
| What is a seizure? | Excessive firing of cortical neurons leading to neurologic symptoms |
| What is the single most useful test to evaluate seizures? | Electroencephalogram (EEG) |
| What tests should be done on a patient suspected to have had a seizure? | Complete neurologic examination. Check for signs of incontinence, tongue lacerations, other injuries to the body to distinguish from syncope. Also check the following laboratory tests: complete blood count (CBC), electrolytes, calcium, glucose, oxygen level, liver function tests, blood urea nitrogen (BUN), creatinine (CR), rapid plasma reagin (RPR), erythrocyte sedimentation rate (ESR), urine toxicology screen. MRI and CT can also be done to rule out a mass. |
| What factors can increase the risk of having a seizure? | History of having a seizure in the past, central nervous system (CNS) tumor, CNS infection, trauma, stroke, high fever in children, drugs |
| What is Todd paralysis?  | Postictal state in which there are focal neurologic deficits that last 24-48 hours; usually associated with focal seizures |

*Prolactin level*

| | |
|---|---|
| Name the two types of generalized seizures. | 1. Tonic-clonic seizures<br>2. Absence seizures |
| Name the seizure disorder described below: | |
| Seizure that may involve motor, autonomic, or sensory functions with no loss of consciousness | Simple partial seizure |
| Elevated prolactin level in postictal state | Tonic-clonic seizure |
| Seizure that arises from one distinct region of the brain | Focal seizure |
| Most commonly involves the temporal lobe | Complex partial seizure |
| Also known as petit mal seizures | Absence seizures |
| Seizure involving both hemispheres with a loss of consciousness and postictal confusion | Generalized seizure |
| Loss of consciousness followed by muscle contractions and then symmetric jerking of extremities | Tonic-clonic seizures |
| Seizures lasting >30 seconds or repetitive seizures lasting >5 minutes with continuous altered level of consciousness | Status epilepticus |
| Often mimics "daydreaming" in children | Absence seizure |
| Associated with cyanosis and urinary incontinence | Tonic-clonic seizure |
| Seizure in which patient has an altered level of consciousness with auditory or visual hallucinations as well as repetitive motor actions and postictal confusion | Complex partial seizures |
| Also known as grand mal seizure | Tonic-clonic seizure |
| Can be caused by electrolyte imbalances, withdrawal from drugs or alcohol, infection (often in CNS), trauma | Status epilepticus |
| Impaired consciousness lasting only a few seconds | Absence seizures |
| EEG with three per second spike and wave | Absence seizure |

**Indicate the treatment for each of the following types of seizures:**

Focal

Phenytoin, carbamazepine, valproic acid

Tonic-clonic

Phenytoin, carbamazepine, phenobarbital

Absence

Ethosuximide and valproic acid

Status epilepticus

This is a medical emergency. Start with the ABCs (airway, breathing, circulation). Benzodiazepine as well as loading dose of phenytoin administration are the next step in treatment, followed by intravenous (IV) sedatives (such as phenobarbital) if patient continues to seize.

**What is the most significant side effect(s) of each of the following antiseizure medications?**

Phenytoin

Agranulocytosis, gingival hyperplasia, hirsutism

Valproic acid

Hepatotoxic; thrombocytopenia; neutropenia

Carbamazepine

Aplastic anemia

**When can antiseizure medication be discontinued in a patient with a history of seizures?**

No seizures for 2 years

# MENINGITIS

**What is the most common bacterial pathogen causing meningitis in adults?**

*Streptococcus pneumoniae* causes up to 60% of meningitis cases.

**What two bacterial pathogens cause most cases of meningitis in young adults?**

*S pneumoniae* and **Neisseria meningitides**

**In what population does Group B Streptococcus cause meningitis?**

Neonates (most common cause of meningitis in neonates)

**What three bacterial pathogens most commonly cause meningitis in neonates?**

1. *Listeria*
2. Group B *Streptococcus* (GBS)
3. *Escherichia coli*

In what adult population does *Listeria* cause meningitis?

Immunocompromised patients

What bacterial pathogen known to cause meningitis is now vaccinated against?

*Haemophilus influenza*

What is the treatment for each of the bacterial pathogens in meningitis?

See Table 4-1.

**Table 4-1** Meningitis Organisms and Treatments

| Organism | Treatment |
| --- | --- |
| S pneumonia | Cefotaxime + vancomycin or ceftriaxone |
| N meningitidis | Penicillin G or ceftriaxone |
| Listeria | Ampicillin (consider adding gentamicin) |
| Group B Streptococcus | Ampicillin |
| H influenzae | Cefotaxime |

What are the classic symptoms of meningitis?

Fever, headache with neck stiffness, photophobia, meningismus, Kernig sign, Brudzinski sign

What is meningismus?

Patient has difficulty touching their chin to their chest.

What is Kernig sign?

Patient has pain when extending the knee with the thigh at 90°.

What is Brudzinski sign?

Neck flexion causes involuntary flexion at the hip and knees.

What test is used to diagnose meningitis?

Lumbar puncture with cerebrospinal fluid (CSF) analysis including Gram stain, cultures

What would the CSF findings be in *bacterial* meningitis (see Table 4-2)?

Increased protein, decreased glucose, very elevated WBCs, elevated opening pressure, and elevated number of neutrophils

What would the CSF findings be in *viral* meningitis?

Normal protein and glucose, elevated WBC, normal or elevated opening pressure, increased lymphocytes

| What would the CSF findings be in *fungal* meningitis? | Elevated protein, decreased glucose, elevated WBC, elevated opening pressure, increased lymphocytes (Table 4-2) |

**Table 4-2** CSF Findings in Meningitis

| Etiology | Protein | Glucose | WBC | Pressure | Differential |
|----------|---------|---------|-----|----------|--------------|
| Bacterial | ↑ | ↓ | ↑ | ↑ | ↑ Neutrophils |
| Viral | Normal | Normal | ↑ | Normal/↑ | ↑ Lymphocytes |
| TB/fungal | ↑ | ↓ | ↑ | ↑ | ↑ Lymphocytes |

KEY

| What is the appropriate empiric treatment for meningitis in each of the following populations? | (see Table 4-3) |

Neonates

1-3 months

Young adults

Adults

Elderly, immunocompromised

**Table 4-3** Meningitis Treatment by Population

| Population | Most Common Organisms | Treatment |
|------------|-----------------------|-----------|
| Neonates (<1 month) | Group B *Streptococcus*; *Listeria*; *E coli* | Cefotaxime + ampicillin |
| 1-3 months | *S pneumoniae*; *H influenzae*; *N meningitidis* | Cefotaxime |
| Children; young adults; crowded living environments | *S pneumoniae*; *N meningitidis* | Ceftriaxone + vancomycin |
| Adults | *S pneumoniae* | Cefotaxime + vancomycin |
| Elderly; immunocompromised | *S pneumoniae*; *Listeria* | Ceftriaxone + ampicillin + vancomycin |

# BRAIN TUMORS

| | |
|---|---|
| What is the most common type of brain tumor? | Metastatic tumor |
| From what primary tumors do most metastatic brain tumors originate? | Lung cancer, breast cancer, melanoma, gastrointestinal (GI) tumors |
| Anatomically, where do most *adult* brain tumors tend to present? | Supratentorially |
| Anatomically, where do most *childhood* brain tumors tend to present? | Infratentorially |
| What are some common symptoms of brain tumors? | Headache (especially upon waking), vomiting, seizures, focal neurologic symptoms |
| How is a brain tumor diagnosed? | CT with contrast/MRI with gadolinium localizes the lesion and a biopsy is used to get the histologic class of the tumor. |
| What is the most common type of primary brain neoplasm? | Astrocytoma |
| What is the most common type of astrocytoma? | Glioblastoma multiforme |
| What is the prognosis of glioblastoma multiforme? | Poor prognosis. 5-year survival is <5%. |
| Where do ependymomas usually arise? | In the fourth ventricle |
| In what population are ependymomas most common? | Children |
| What is the prognosis? | 80% 5-year survival |
| What is the most common cranial nerve tumor? | Schwannoma |
| What cranial nerve does a schwannoma affect? | Cranial nerve VIII—vestibular division |
| What is the most common mesodermal tumor? | Meningioma |

| | |
|---|---|
| How are most brain tumors treated? | Surgical excision and radiation. Medulloblastomas also require chemotherapy and schwannomas are treated with surgery alone. |

# DEMYELINATING DISEASES

| | |
|---|---|
| What is the most common demyelinating disorder? | Multiple sclerosis (MS) |
| Who is at higher risk for developing MS? | Those with a family history of MS, those who lived up until puberty in northern latitudes or temperate climates, female sex (incidence is 2:1 female:male) |
| What age is the peak age of MS presentation? | Age 20-40 |
| What is the typical course of the disease? | Multiple progressive neurologic alterations that wax and wane and cannot be explained by a single lesion |
| What are some of the signs and symptoms of MS? | Limb weakness, paresthesias, optic neuritis, **nystagmus, scanning speech, intranuclear ophthalmoplegia,** vertigo, diplopia |
| What is Lhermitte sign? | Shock-like sensation down the spine when patient flexes their neck. Also known as the "barber chair phenomenon." |
| What can be seen on MRI on a patient with MS? | MRI shows multiple, asymmetric, periventricular plaques with multiple areas of demyelination. |
| What does the CSF show in an MS patient? | Oligoclonal bands; elevated IgG |
| What is the treatment for MS? | Steroids during acute episodes and interferon-β to prolong remission |
| What is the other name for amyotrophic lateral sclerosis (ALS)? | Lou Gehrig disease |

| | |
|---|---|
| What is the underlying pathology in ALS? | Slowly progressive loss of upper and lower motor neurons in the CNS |
| What are the clinical signs and symptoms of ALS? | Asymmetric, progressive muscle weakness initially with fasciculations which present clinically as difficulty swallowing. Patients also have upper motor neuron and lower motor neuron signs on physical examination. They do not have bowel or bladder involvement. |
| Give examples of both upper and lower motor neuron signs? | Upper motor neuron signs: spastic paralysis, hyperreflexia, upgoing Babinski<br><br>Lower motor neuron signs: flaccid paralysis, fasciculations, absent Babinski |
| How is ALS diagnosed? | Clinically there should be a combination of upper motor neuron and lower motor neuron symptoms in three or more extremities. An electromyogram (EMG) will show widespread denervation and fibrillation potentials in at least three limbs. |
| What is the main treatment for ALS? | Supportive care |
| What do ALS patients ultimately die from? | Respiratory failure |
| What is Guillain-Barré syndrome? | An autoimmune, acute demyelinating disorder affecting the **peripheral nerves** (particularly motor fibers) |
| What bacterial infection is Guillain-Barré syndrome associated with? | *Campylobacter jejuni* |
| What often precedes Guillain-Barré syndrome? | A bacterial infection causing diarrhea, specifically with *Campylobacter*, viral infection, or vaccination |
| Clinically, how does Guillain-Barré syndrome present? | **Symmetric ascending paralysis**. Symptoms usually begin with distal weakness and progress to proximal weakness with hyporeflexia and facial diplegia. It can eventually progress to paralysis of the diaphragm, leading to respiratory failure. |

| | |
|---|---|
| What tests would you do to diagnose Guillain-Barré syndrome? | Lumbar puncture and EMG |
| What would you see in the CSF after a lumbar puncture? | ↑ ↑ protein; normal cell count—this is known as **albuminocytologic dissociation** |
| What interventions should be undertaken in a patient with Guillain-Barré syndrome? | Monitor respiratory function very closely and **intubate** if needed. Medical treatment includes plasmapheresis and intravenous immunoglobulin (IVIG). |
| What is the prognosis? | Good prognosis |

## COGNITIVE DISORDERS

| | |
|---|---|
| What is dementia? | A syndrome of global intellectual and cognitive deficits which are constant and progressive. Patients have no sensory abnormalities (no auditory or visual hallucinations) |
| What specific type of cognitive deficit is dementia usually characterized by? | Memory loss (Remember: dememtia) |
| What types of cognitive impairments characterize dementia? | Impairments in memory, abstract thought, planning and organization as well as aphasia, apraxia, and agnosia |
| What are the causes of dementia? | Alzheimer; Parkinson, Huntington; seizure disorder; stroke; $B_{12}$ deficiency; thiamine deficiency; folate deficiency; alcoholism; head trauma (especially repetitive); neurotoxins; CNS infections such as syphilis; CNS malignancies; normal pressure hydrocephalus |
| | Degenerative disorders (Alzheimer, Parkinson, Huntington) (Remember the mnemonic: **DEMENTIAS**) |
| | Electrolyte imbalances/Endocrine |
| | Mass effect |
| | Epilepsy |
| | Neurotoxins |
| | Trauma |
| | Infection |
| | Alzheimer is most common (70%-80%) |
| | Stroke |

**What tests would you order if you suspected dementia in a patient?**

Head CT, CBC, electrolytes, BUN, creatinine, AST, ALT, $B_{12}$, folate, rapid plasma region (RPR), thyroid-stimulating hormone (TSH), urine toxicology screen

**What medical problem can mimic dementia?**

Depression can present as pseudodementia.

**What class of medications should be avoided in demented patients?**

Benzodiazepines

**What is the general treatment for dementia?**

Treat underlying cause if one is found, otherwise supportive treatment. Patients should also learn to use environmental clues.

**What is delirium?**

Sudden and transient global cognitive deficits that **wax and wane**

**What specific clinical symptom distinguishes delirium from dementia?**

Patients with delirium have sensory deficits which include **auditory and visual hallucinations**.

**What are the symptoms of delirium?**

**Waxing and waning levels of consciousness and sensory disturbances.** Patients are often found to be anxious, combative, have poor memory, and have decreased attention span.

**What are the main etiologies of delirium?**

Remember the mnemonic **HIDE:**

Hypoxia

Infection

Drugs

Electrolyte abnormalities

**What tests would you order if you suspected delirium?**

CBC, electrolytes, glucose, BUN, creatinine, AST, ALT, TSH, thiamine, B12, urinalysis, chest x-ray (CXR), urine toxicology screen, pulse oximetry, possibly a head CT

**What else would be very important to examine in a patient with delirium?**

Patient's medication list

**What two-drug classes are often found to cause delirium?**

1. Anticholinergics
2. Benzodiazepines

| | |
|---|---|
| What is the most common infection leading to delirium in the elderly? | Urinary tract infection (UTI) |
| What is the main treatment for delirium? | Treat the underlying cause. Antipsychotics can be used to help control symptoms. |
| How can dementia be distinguished from delirium? | See Table 4-4. |

**Table 4-4** Characteristics of Dementia Vs Delirium

| Dementia | Delirium |
|---|---|
| Constant cognitive deficits which are progressive over time | **Waxing and waning** of cognitive deficits (usually worse at night) called **"sundowning"** |
| No audio/visual hallucinations | Hallucinations common |
| Deficits are irreversible | Deficits can be reversed if insulting factors removed |
| No alteration in the level of consciousness | Altered level of consciousness |

| | |
|---|---|
| What is the most common cause of dementia? | Alzheimer |
| What is found in the cerebral cortex in patients with Alzheimer? | **Amyloid plaques and neurofibrillary tangles** |
| What is the most common symptom of Alzheimer? | Memory deficits |
| What can be seen on CT in a patient with Alzheimer? | Cortical atrophy |
| What genotype is Alzheimer associated with? | Apolipoprotein E |
| How can Alzheimer be diagnosed? | It is a clinical diagnosis because it can only be diagnosed definitively at autopsy. |
| What medications can slow the cognitive decline in Alzheimer? | Anticholinesterase inhibitors: donepezil (Aricept), tacrine |

What is the underlying pathology in Parkinson disease?

Degeneration of dopaminergic neurons in the **substantia nigra**

What are the pathognomonic symptoms of Parkinson disease?

**Cogwheel rigidity, resting tremor, bradykinesia, shuffling gait, mask-like faces, postural instability**

What are the treatment options for Parkinson disease?

Amantadine; Sinemet (levodopa/carbidopa); benztropine, selegiline, bromocriptine

What is the mechanism of amantadine and what symptom is it best for?

Blocks dopamine reuptake in presynaptic neurons and treats **bradykinesia** mainly in mild disease

What is the mechanism of Sinemet and what symptom does it best treat?

Sinemet is a combination of levadopa and carbidopa. Levodopa is converted into dopamine in the substantia nigra. Carbidopa is necessary because it cannot cross the blood-brain barrier and prevents levodopa metabolism by peripheral tissues. It is also best for treating bradykinesia.

Name some of the anticholinergic drugs.

Benztropine, trihexyphenidyl

What symptom of Parkinson disease do anticholinergics best treat?

Tremor

What is the mechanism of selegiline?

Monoamine oxidase (MAO) inhibitor which blocks dopamine metabolism

What is the mechanism of bromocriptine?

Dopamine agonist

What kind of genetic pattern does Huntington disease follow?

Autosomal dominant

On what chromosome is the genetic alteration found and what is the genetic defect?

Chromosome 4; triple repeat of CAG

In what age range does Huntington disease usually present?

Between 30 and 50 years of age

What is the underlying pathophysiology of Huntington disease?

Atrophy of the caudate nucleus

What are the typical signs and symptoms of Huntington disease? | Choreiform movements, dementia, **schizophreniform changes**, ataxic gait

What is the treatment for Huntington disease? | Supportive treatment. Antipsychotics can be used as needed for psychotic symptoms.

What is the problem in Wilson disease? | Defect in copper metabolism

What are the symptoms of Wilson disease? | Tremors and rigidity as well as psychiatric changes such as schizophrenia, manic depression; patients have parkinsonian features

What is the pathognomonic physical examination finding in Wilson disease? | **Kayser-Fleischer ring around the cornea**

How is Wilson disease diagnosed? | Elevated serum ceruloplasmin

What is the treatment for Wilson disease? | Penicillamine with pyridoxine (vitamin $B_6$) and zinc. Liver transplantation is the final treatment if patient fails medical therapy.

## HEADACHE

What is the most common type of headache? | Tension headache

What are signs and symptoms of a tension headache? | Bilateral, band-like, dull, most intense at neck/occiput, worsened with stress

What psychiatric disorder is it most commonly associated with? | Depression

What is the most common age group with this type of headache? | Between 20 and 50 years of age

What type of headache is characterized by rhinorrhea, being unilateral, stabbing, retro-orbital pain, ipsilateral lacrimation, ptosis, and nasal congestion? | Cluster headache

| | |
|---|---|
| What type of headache is characterized by photophobia, nausea, aura, and being unilateral? | Migraine headache |
| What are some common triggers for migraines? | Menstruation, stress, foods, alcohol |
| What type of headache is associated with jaw claudicating? | Temporal arteritis (usually a unilateral temporal headache with temporal artery tenderness) |
| What is the predilection for temporal arteritis? | Female > male |
| What are the risks of temporal arteritis? | Optic neuritis and blindness if not treated |
| What is it associated with? | Polymyalgia rheumatica |
| How is it diagnosed? | Must do a temporal artery biopsy; elevated ESR is just a screening test |
| What is the treatment for temporal arteritis? | High-dose steroids |

## INTRACRANIAL BLEEDING

| | |
|---|---|
| What is "the worst headache of my life"? | Subarachnoid hemorrhage (SAH) |
| What is the most common cause of SAH? | Head trauma |
| What is the most common underlying cause of a spontaneous SAH? | Aneurysm rupture |
| What is the most common heritable disorder associated with SAH? | Autosomal dominant polycystic kidney disease |
| How is an SAH diagnosed? | CT scan shows subarachnoid blood (dark); lumbar puncture shows bloody CSF with xanthochromia; cerebral angiography can be done to find berry aneurysms. |
| What is the immediate treatment for an SAH? | ICU admission. Goal is to decrease intracranial pressure (ICP). Give nimodipine to decrease chance of vasospasm by controlling blood pressure, raise the head of the bed, and administer IV fluids as needed. |

What is the second-line treatment for an SAH?

Surgical evacuation of blood via burr holes

What is a berry aneurysm?

Outpouching of vessels in the circle of Willis, usually at bifurcations (looks like a berry)

What medical condition is a berry aneurism associated with?

Polycystic kidney disease, Marfan disease

What is a symptom of berry aneurysm rupture?

Third nerve palsy

What is the most common location for a berry aneurysm?

Anterior communicating artery (30%), followed by posterior communicating artery, then middle cerebral artery

What type of hemorrhage is associated with a lateral skull fracture?

Epidural hematoma

What artery is involved in an epidural hematoma?

Middle meningeal artery

What is the sequence of events in an epidural hematoma?

The patient has a lucid interval lasting from minutes to hours followed by a loss of consciousness and hemiparesis.

What can cause a "blown" pupil in a patient with an epidural hematoma?

Uncal herniation

What is seen on CT in a patient with an epidural hematoma?

Convex (lens shaped) hyperdensity that does not cross the midline

What is the treatment for an epidural hematoma?

Surgical evacuation of the hematoma via burr holes

What vessels are involved in a subdural hemorrhage?

Bridging veins

In what population are subdural hematomas most common?

The elderly and alcoholics

What is the course of events in a subdural hematoma?

Patient can have symptoms similar to dementia since mental status changes and hemiparesis can present subacutely.

What is seen on CT in a patient with a subdural hematoma?

Crescent-shaped, concave hyperdensity that may cross the midline

# VERTIGO

What type of vertigo is characterized by horizontal nystagmus?

Peripheral vertigo

What type of vertigo is characterized by vertical nystagmus?

Central vertigo

What is the most common cause of vertigo?

Benign positional vertigo

What are the signs of benign positional vertigo?

Sudden, episodic vertigo that occurs with quick head movement and lasts for seconds

How is benign positional vertigo diagnosed?

Dix-Hallpike maneuver—From a sitting position, the physician turns the patients head 45° to the right as the patient lies back to the supine position. After 30 seconds the patient is returned to the sitting position and observed. Vertigo with or without nystagmus is a positive test.

What is the treatment of benign positional vertigo?

Epley maneuvers

What is the etiology of Meniere disease?

Excess endolymph causes dilation of the membranous labyrinth

What is the triad of symptoms?

1. Tinnitus
2. Hearing loss
3. Episodic vertigo lasting **hours**

What does audiometry show in Meniere disease?

Low-frequency pure-tone hearing loss

What is the treatment for Meniere disease?

Low salt intake and acetazolamide. If acute, you could use antihistamines, anticholinergics, or antiemetics. Surgery may be necessary.

What type of vertigo follows a viral respiratory illness?

Viral labyrinthitis

How long does the vertigo last?          Days to weeks

What is the treatment for viral          Meclizine
labyrinthitis?

# CLINICAL VIGNETTES

A 64-year-old male smoker with past medical history of hypertension, hyperlipidemia, and type 2 diabetes presents to the ER with a right-sided facial droop as well as weakness of the right arm and leg. Symptoms began about 3 hours prior. The patient currently takes aspirin 81 mg as a part of his daily regimen. What is this patient's strongest modifiable risk factor for his current condition?

Hypertension

A 22-year-old female patient with no past medical history comes to your office complaining of increased "fatigue" particularly with repeated effort of muscle use or activity. She has noticed that her vision is blurry lately and that her eye lids seem to be droopy. You examine her and find that her muscle strength seems to deteriorate with repeated efforts. Sensation is normal. What condition do you initially suspect?

Myasthenia gravis

A 36-year-old male with a past medical history of psoriasis comes in complaining of "dizziness." He is particularly dizzy and nauseous when he lies in bed and turns his head from left to right. He denies any tinnitus or hearing loss or any other neurologic symptoms. You suspect he has benign positional vertigo. What physical examination test could help with this diagnosis?

Dix-Hallpike maneuver

An 85-year-old female presents to your office complaining of new-onset headache over the past month. Headache tends to be on the left side only. She denies any problems with her vision. She has no photophobia with headaches nor is she bothered by sound. On review of symptoms she does complain of some jaw pain. What condition should be ruled out in this case?

Temporal arteritis

A 76-year-old female who lives in a retirement community is admitted for an UTI. In the evening time, the patient becomes combative and disoriented. What is the most likely diagnosis?

Delirium

# CHAPTER 5

# Gastroenterology

## ESOPHAGEAL DISORDERS

| | |
|---|---|
| What is dysphagia? | Difficulty swallowing |
| What is odynophagia? | Pain with swallowing |
| How does oropharyngeal dysphagia present? | More difficulty initiating the swallowing of liquids than solids |
| How does esophageal dysphagia present in terms of swallowing? | Difficulty swallowing both liquids and solids |
| What are the causes of oropharyngeal dysphagia? | Neurologic disorders (muscular, cranial nerve diseases), Zenker diverticulum, thyromegaly, sphincter dysfunction, oropharyngeal cancers |
| What is a Zenker diverticulum? | Lower pharyngeal outpouching of the muscular wall. Pulsion diverticulum secondary to pressure from swallowing. |
| What are the signs and symptoms of Zenker diverticulum? | Halitosis, neck mass on the left, dysphagia, aspiration |
| How is Zenker diverticulum diagnosed? | Clinical palpation of a left-sided neck mass or a barium swallow |
| What is the treatment for Zenker diverticulum? | Cricopharyngeal myotomy or surgical excision |
| What are the causes of esophageal dysphagia? | 1. Mechanical obstruction: esophageal cancer, Schatzki ring, peptic stricture<br>2. Problem with esophageal motility: achalasia, diffuse esophageal spasm, or scleroderma |

How do symptoms of mechanical dysphagia differ from dysphagia secondary to motility problems?

Patients with mechanical dysphagia have more difficulty with solids than liquids whereas motility disorders cause difficulty with both solids and liquids.

What is the most common motility disorder often seen in patients with scleroderma?

Esophageal hypomotility

What defines achalasia?

Loss of esophageal peristalsis with an inability of the lower esophageal sphincter to relax due to ganglionic loss of **Auerbach plexus**.

What is the diagnostic feature seen on barium swallow in a patient with achalasia?

"Bird's beak" appearance (dilation of the proximal esophagus with narrowing of the distal esophagus)

What would manometry demonstrate in a patient with achalasia?

Increased pressure at the lower esophageal sphincter with no relaxation with swallowing

How is achalasia treated?

Balloon dilatation, sphincter myotomy, local botulinum toxin

What is the diagnostic feature seen on barium swallow in a patient with diffuse esophageal spasm?

"Corkscrew pattern"

What is the treatment for diffuse esophageal spasm?

Nitroglycerin, calcium channel blockers

What is Schatzki ring?

Narrowing of the lower esophageal ring

What is Plummer-Vinson syndrome?

Esophageal webs, atrophic glossitis, and dysphagia associated with iron deficiency anemia

# GASTROESOPHAGEAL REFLUX DISEASE

What are the underlying causes of gastroesophageal reflux disease (GERD)?

Incompetent lower esophageal sphincter, obesity, hiatal hernia, pregnancy, decreased esophageal motility, delayed gastric emptying

What are the signs and symptoms of GERD?

Postprandial epigastric (chest) burning worse in supine position, cough, hoarse voice, regurgitation

How is GERD diagnosed?

It is a clinical diagnosis.

| What is the treatment for GERD? | First-line treatment is lifestyle modification; weight loss; avoidance of instigating foods such as caffeine, fatty foods; avoid eating right before going to sleep |
| --- | --- |
| | Second-line treatment: H2 blockers |
| | Third-line treatment: If H2 blockers fail, try proton pump inhibitors (PPIs) |
| | Last resort: Nissen fundoplication |
| What can be the long-term effects of chronic GERD? | Barrett esophagus, peptic stricture, and esophageal cancer |
| What is Barrett esophagus? | Transformation of normal squamous epithelium to columnar epithelium |
| What is the risk with Barrett esophagus? | 10% lifetime risk of transforming into esophageal adenocarcinoma |

## GASTRITIS

| What is gastritis? | Inflammation of the gastric mucosa |
| --- | --- |

Name the type of gastritis that matches the statement below:

| Gastritis most likely to be found in the fundus | Type A |
| --- | --- |
| Gastritis most likely to be found in the antrum of the stomach | Type B |
| Associated with autoimmune causes, achlorhydria, pernicious anemia | **Type A** |
| Most common cause is nonsteroidal anti-inflammatory drug (NSAID) use | Type B |
| Can be caused by *Helicobacter pylori* infection | Type B |
| Associated with risk for peptic ulcer disease and gastric cancer | Type B |

| What are the signs and symptoms of gastritis? | May be asymptomatic; otherwise symptoms are epigastric pain, weight loss, nausea, vomiting, hematemesis, **coffee ground emesis** |
| --- | --- |

How is gastritis diagnosed?

Endoscopy

What is the treatment for gastritis?

It depends on the etiology.

If caused by *H pylori*—triple therapy with PPI, two antibiotics, and bismuth compound

If caused by NSAID use—discontinue NSAID use; start sucralfate, PPI, or H2 blocker

If caused by post-procedure, hospitalization stress—intravenous (IV) H2 blocker

If caused by pernicious anemia— vitamin $B_{12}$ treatment

# PEPTIC ULCERS

What are the two types of peptic ulcers?

1. Duodenal ulcer
2. Gastric ulcer

Which type of ulcer is more common?

Duodenal ulcers are twice as common.

What is the underlying pathology in a patient with a duodenal ulcer?

Most have increased acid production.

How does the underlying pathology of gastric ulcers differ from that of duodenal ulcers?

Gastric ulcers are not caused by increased acid production. Patients are more likely to have decreased mucosal protection.

What bacterial infection is found in 90% of patients with duodenal ulcers?

*H pylori*

What percentage of gastric ulcers are associated with *H pylori* infection?

70%

What test can determine if a patient may be infected with *H pylori*?

Stool *H pylori* antigen, urea breath test, serum IgG test

What is the drawback of the *H pylori* blood test?

It does not indicate an **active** infection. It will be positive even if the patient was infected in the past and is not currently infected. The test also has a low sensitivity.

| | |
|---|---|
| **What are the two most common causes of peptic ulcer disease?** | 1. *H pylori* infection<br>2. Frequent NSAID use |
| **What are the risk factors for a peptic ulcer?** | Smoking, significant alcohol use, frequent NSAID use, significant physiologic stress (examples are surgery, trauma, burns), and hypersecretory states |
| **Name three hypersecretory states.** | 1. Zollinger-Ellison syndrome<br>2. Multiple endocrine neoplasia type I (MEN I)<br>3. Antral G-cell hyperplasia |
| **What are the signs and symptoms of a duodenal ulcer?** | Burning epigastric pain that is usually 2-3 hours postprandially; relieved by food or antacids; pain may radiate to the back; pain awakens patient at night; nausea and sometimes vomiting; hematemesis/melena if patient has a gastrointestinal (GI) bleed |
| **What are the signs and symptoms of a gastric ulcer?** | Same as that for a duodenal ulcer except that pain is greater with meals, so patients often lose weight |
| **What tests would you order if you suspected a peptic ulcer?** | Complete blood count (CBC) to make sure patient is not anemic; upper GI endoscopy or upper GI series; *H pylori* screening |
| **What should be ruled out in a patient with a gastric ulcer?** | Malignancy |
| **How can malignancy be ruled out?** | A biopsy of the ulcerated region should be done during endoscopy |
| **What is a gastric ulcer in a burn patient called?** | **Curling ulcer** |
| **What is a gastric ulcer in a patient with central nervous system (CNS) damage called?** | **Cushing ulcer** |
| **How is peptic ulcer disease treated?** | Avoidance of instigating factors such as smoking and NSAIDs; H2 blockers or PPIs, mucosal protectors such as bismuth, and antibiotics if the patient is infected with *H pylori* |

How is an *H pylori* infection treated?

**Triple therapy:** PPI + bismuth compound + two antibiotics for 14 days For example: omeprazole + amoxicillin (or metronidazole) + clarithromycin + bismuth compound

What are some complications of peptic ulcer disease?

Hemorrhage, obstruction, perforation

When would you suspect a perforated duodenal ulcer?

Severe epigastric pain that radiates to the back

What studies would you order if you suspected a perforated ulcer?

Abdominal series or upper GI series with contrast **(do not use barium)**

What would you expect to see on an abdominal series if there was a perforated ulcer?

Free air under the diaphragm

What is the treatment for a perforated ulcer?

Npo (nothing by mouth), IV fluids, antibiotics, emergent surgery

What are the typical symptoms of gastric outlet obstruction?

Nausea, vomiting, weight loss, distended abdomen, loud bowel sounds

What is the most serious complication of a posterior duodenal ulcer?

Erosion into the gastroduodenal artery can lead to a massive hemorrhage.

What symptoms could be a red flag for a gastric malignancy?

Early satiety with weight loss

What are the risk factors for gastric cancer?

Diets with high nitrosamines or salt content, history of chronic gastritis, low-fiber diets, gastric ulcer, smoking, blood group A, Japanese ethnicity

What blood group type is more likely to develop gastric cancer?

Type A

In what part of the stomach is gastric cancer usually found?

In the antrum of the stomach

What is the most common type of gastric cancer?

Adenocarcinoma

Name the physical findings associated
with metastatic gastric cancer
described below:

    Palpable left supraclavicular          Virchow node
    lymph node

    Hard lymph nodule palpable at the    Sister Mary Joseph sign
    umbilicus

    Palpable ovarian mass that           Krukenberg tumor
    originates from the metastasis of
    signet-ring cells

    Lymph node that can be palpated     Blumer shelf
    on a rectal examination due to
    metastasis to the pouch of Douglas

What is the most fatal form of gastric    Linitis plastica (diffusely infiltrating
cancer?                           gastric cancer)

# GI BLEED

What are signs of an upper GI bleed?   Hematemesis, coffee ground emesis,
                                 melena (black, tarry stools), bright red
                                 blood per rectum (BRBPR) only if the
                                 bleed is very brisk

What are the six main causes of upper  Remember the mnemonic **PAGE ME!**
GI bleeds?                        1.  Peptic ulcer
                       2.  Atrioventricular (AV) malformation
                       3.  Gastritis
                       4.  Esophageal varices
                       5.  Mallory-Weiss tear
                       6.  Esophagitis

What is a Mallory-Weiss tear?     Small esophageal tear usually near the
                                 gastroesophageal (GE) junction that is
                                 caused by vomiting or retching

What blood tests would you order in a  CBC (look for anemia, platelet
patient you thought may have a GI    abnormality), blood urea nitrogen
bleed?                        (BUN) (fresh bleeding may lead to
                                 elevated BUN), prothrombin time (PT),
                                 partial thromboplastin time (PTT),
                                 international normalized ratio (INR),
                                 bleeding abnormalities

| | |
|---|---|
| What is the best diagnostic test in a patient with upper GI bleed? | Endoscopy |
| How are bleeding varices treated? | Ligation or injection of vessels with sclerosing or vasoconstrictive agents |
| How should all GI bleeds be treated? | Emergency airway, breathing, circulation (ABCs) as well as IV fluid resuscitation, gastric lavage and nasogastric (NG) tube if needed |
| What are the signs of a lower GI bleed? | BRBPR, maroon or dark red stool, anemia |
| What are the six most common causes of lower GI bleeding? | 1. **Diverticulosis**<br>2. **AV malformation**<br>3. **Hemorrhoids**<br>4. **Colitis**<br>5. **Colon cancer**<br>6. **Colonic polyps** |
| What is the most common cause of a major lower GI bleed in a patient older than 60? | Diverticulosis |
| What physical examination and imaging study would you do on a patient with suspected lower GI bleed? | **Always** do a rectal examination; colonoscopy |
| If no clear source is found, what other studies can be done? | Endoscopy to rule out an upper GI source, tagged red blood cell (RBC) scan; arteriography, gastric lavage; barium enema (but not if there is acute blood loss) |

# COLON

| | |
|---|---|
| What is a true diverticulum? | Colonic herniation involving the full thickness of bowel wall |
| What is a false diverticulum? | Colonic mucosal herniation through the muscular layer which is acquired |
| Which type of diverticulum is more common? | False |

In what part of the colon are diverticula most commonly found?

Sigmoid

What is diverticulosis?

Presence of multiple diverticula in the colon

What is thought to be an important risk factor for the development of diverticulosis?

Low-fiber diet

Why do diverticula bleed?

Diverticula which are inflamed erode through an artery and cause profuse bleeding that usually subsides on its own.

What is the treatment for diverticulosis?

Increase of fiber in diet and decrease of obstructing foods such as seeds and fatty foods

What is diverticulitis?

"-itis" implies inflammation. Diverticulitis is inflammation of a diverticulum secondary to infection.

What is the most common symptom of diverticulitis?

The most common presenting symptom is left **lower quadrant abdominal pain.**

What are other signs and symptoms of diverticulitis?

Constipation, fever, elevated white blood cells (WBCs), bleeding is much less common than with diverticulosis

What are the four serious complications of diverticulitis?

1. Perforation through the bowel wall causing peritonitis
2. Fistula formation
3. Abscess
4. Obstruction

How do patients who develop a colovesicular fistula present?

Multiple urinary tract infections (UTIs)

What is the best imaging test to diagnose diverticulitis?

Computed tomography (CT) of the abdomen and pelvis

What studies are contraindicated in diverticulitis?

Colonoscopy, contrast enema

What is the treatment for diverticulitis?

Npo, IV fluids, antibiotics to cover anaerobes and enteric organisms

| | |
|---|---|
| What is the treatment for recurrent bouts of diverticulitis or severe cases? | Elective sigmoid colectomy |
| How would you treat an abscess secondary to diverticulitis? | CT or ultrasound-guided percutaneous drainage |
| How do you treat obstruction or perforation secondary to diverticulitis? | Surgical resection of affected bowel with a colostomy that is usually temporary |
| What is the most common nosocomial enteric infection? | *Clostridium difficile* |
| What can a *C difficile* infection lead to? | **Pseudomembranous colitis** |
| What antibiotic is classically associated with *C difficile* infection? | **Clindamycin** |
| What are the symptoms of *C difficile* infection? | Diarrhea and abdominal cramping/pain |
| How is a *C difficile* infection diagnosed? | *C difficile* stool toxin, stool leukocytes |
| How is a *C difficile* infection treated? | Stop the offending agent and treat with po metronidazole or vancomycin. |
| How is pseudomembranous colitis confirmed? | On colonoscopy or sigmoidoscopy, a yellow plaque adherent to the colonic mucosa can be seen. |
| What is volvulus? | Twisting of the bowel around the mesenteric base |
| What is the most common location of volvulus? | Sigmoid colon |
| What is the second most common location of volvulus? | Cecum |
| What are the symptoms of a volvulus? | Painful, distended abdomen; high-pitched bowel sounds; tympany on percussion |
| What is the classic sign of volvulus on an abdominal series? | Dilated loops of bowel with a **kidney-bean** appearance |
| What is the sign of volvulus on a barium enema? | Bird's beak appearance with the beak pointing to the area where the rotation has occurred |

**What is the treatment for volvulus?**

Sigmoidoscopy or colonoscopy is usually therapeutic for decompression.

**What is the second most common cancer causing death in the United States?**

Colon cancer

**What are the risk factors for colon cancer?**

Family history

Low-fiber diet

Familial adenomatous polyposis (FAP)

Hereditary nonpolyposis colorectal cancer

High-fat diet

Colonic adenomas

Age >50

Inflammatory bowel disease

**What are the general signs and symptoms of colon cancer?**

Weight loss, fatigue, iron deficiency anemia in a male >50 years of age is colon cancer (CA) until proven otherwise; GI bleed, constipation, distended abdomen secondary to obstruction, pencil-thin stools

**How do the symptoms of right-sided- and left-sided colon cancer differ?**

Left-sided colon cancer presents as constipation.

Right-sided colon cancer presents as anemia secondary to blood loss.

**What are the recommendations for colon cancer screening?**

Starting age 50, a colonoscopy every 10 years or a sigmoidoscopy every 5 years with annual digital rectal and hemoccult examination

**How are the screening recommendations different in patients with a family history of colon cancer?**

Start screening 10 years prior to the age that the family member was diagnosed with cancer.

**How is colon cancer diagnosed?**

Biopsy of the lesion on colonoscopy/ sigmoidoscopy

**What laboratory marker can be used to help follow the progression of colon cancer and its treatments?**

Carcinoembryonic antigen (CEA)—but it cannot be used as a screening test

How is colon cancer staged and what is the prognosis of each stage?

TNM (tumor node metastasis) classification (Tables 5-1A and 5-1B)

**Table 5-1A** Colon Cancer Staging

| Staging of Primary Tumor | Nodal Involvement | Metastasis |
|---|---|---|
| Tis: Carcinoma in situ | N0: No regional node involvement | M0: No metastasis |
| T1: Tumor invades submucosa | N1: Metastasis in one to three regional lymph nodes | M1: Distant metastasis present |
| T2: Tumor invades muscularis propria | N2: Metastasis in four or more regional lymph nodes | |
| T3: Tumor invades the subserosa or into the nonperitoneal pericolic or perirectal tissues | | |
| T4: Tumor perforates the visceral peritoneum or directly invades other organs | | |

**Table 5-1B** Colon Cancer Prognosis Based on Staging

| Stage | | T | N | M | Approximate 5-Year Prognosis |
|---|---|---|---|---|---|
| Stage | 0 | Tis | N0 | M0 | >90% |
| Stage | I | T1 | N0 | M0 | >90% |
| | | T2 | N0 | M0 | |
| Stage | II A | T3 | N0 | M0 | 70%-85% |
| | II B | T4 | N0 | M0 | 55%-65% |
| Stage | III A | T1, T2 | N1 | M0 | 45%-55% |
| | III B | T3, T4 | N1 | M0 | 20%-35% |
| | III C | Any T | N2 | M0 | |
| Stage | IV | Any T | Any N | M1 | <5% |

What is the treatment of colon cancer?

Surgical resection; radiation therapy (if rectal cancer), and chemotherapy for stages B and C

# INFLAMMATORY BOWEL

| | |
|---|---|
| What is ulcerative colitis (UC)? | Inflammatory bowel disease that affects the colon |
| What classic symptom is associated with UC? | **Bloody diarrhea** |
| What other serious symptom can sometimes occur with UC? | Toxic megacolon |
| Where are lesions found in UC? | Large intestine only |
| Where do the lesions usually first appear? | Rectum |
| How do lesions spread in UC? | Proximally from the rectum |
| How is UC diagnosed? | Colonoscopy with biopsy |
| What is seen on colonoscopic biopsy in a patient with UC? | **Crypt abscess**; distorted cells |
| How is the mucosa of the colon described in a patient with UC? | Friable mucosa with erosions and erythema |
| On biopsy, what is the depth of involvement of the lesions? | Mucosa and submucosa only |
| What is ulcerative proctitis? | A subtype of UC in which only the rectum is involved |
| What is the treatment for each of the following severities of UC: | |
| Distal colitis (mild) | **Mesalamine** |
| Moderate colitis | Mesalamine + **sulfasalazine ±** corticosteroids |
| Severe colitis | IV corticosteroids + azathioprine ; resistant cases try Remicade; unresponsive cases require resection |
| Fulminant colitis? | Broad-spectrum antibiotics, surgery |
| What is Crohn disease? | Inflammatory bowel disease that affects the GI tract; there could be an infectious etiology |

| | |
|---|---|
| What part of the GI tract can Crohn disease involve? | From the mouth to the rectum, but often with rectal sparing |
| What is the classic symptom of Crohn disease? | **Bloody or watery diarrhea** (although the diarrhea does not always have to be bloody) |
| What are some other physical examination findings in Crohn disease? | Fistulas, fissures, fever, abdominal pain |
| How is Crohn disease diagnosed? | Colonoscopy and biopsy |
| How are the lesions classically spread in Crohn disease? | There are **skip lesions,** which means that there is no contiguous spread. The lesions are disseminated through the entire colon. |
| What is the depth of the lesions on biopsy? | Lesions go through all layers—they are **transmural**. |
| On physical examination, what type of lesion is often found in the mouth of a patient with Crohn disease? | Aphthous ulcer |
| What is the mnemonic to remember Crohn disease? | The old, **Crohn skipped** over the **cobblestone**. |
| What is the treatment for Crohn disease? | Sulfasalazine, corticosteroids; for unresponsive patients, try mercaptopurine, azathioprine, infliximab |
| What are the differences between UC and Crohn disease? | See Table 5-2. |

**Table 5-2** Crohn Disease Vs Ulcerative Colitis

| Crohn Disease | Ulcerative Colitis |
|---|---|
| Lesions in small and large intestine | Lesions only in large intestine |
| Rectal involvement uncommon | Rectal involvement common |
| Transmural | Submucosa/mucosa only |
| Skip lesions | Lesions are contiguous |
| Fissures and fistulas common | No fissures or fistulas |
| Lower risk for colon cancer | High risk for colon cancer |

| | |
|---|---|
| Name six extraintestinal manifestations of both UC and Crohn disease? | 1. Erythema nodosum<br>2. Pyoderma gangrenosum<br>3. Uveitis<br>4. **Ankylosing spondylitis**<br>5. Primary sclerosing cholangitis<br>6. Arthritis |

# DIARRHEA

| | |
|---|---|
| What is the definition of diarrhea? | Daily stool weighing >200 g |
| What are the most common causes of bacterial and parasitic bloody diarrhea? | Remember the mnemonic **whY CaSES**:<br>*Yersinia*<br>*Campylobacter*, cholera<br>*Shigella*<br>*Escherichia coli, Entamoeba histolytica*<br>*Salmonella* |
| What is the treatment for bacterial bloody diarrhea? | Ciprofloxacin or bactrim |
| What are viral causes of bloody diarrhea? | Rotavirus and Norwalk virus |
| What is the treatment for bloody diarrhea caused by a virus? | IV fluids |
| What is the treatment for parasitic bloody diarrhea? | Metronidazole |
| What studies would you order in a patient with bloody diarrhea? | CBC, stool for ova and parasites, stool for fecal leukocytes, stool culture |
| What acid-base disorder can you expect to see in a patient with severe diarrhea? | Metabolic acidosis |

# MALABSORPTION DISORDERS

Name the malabsorption disorder
described below:

| | |
|---|---|
| Gluten-induced enteropathy | Celiac sprue |
| Caused by tropical infection | Tropical sprue |
| Protein-losing enteropathy with large gastric folds seen on barium swallow | Menetrier disease |
| Most common malabsorptive disorder of adulthood | Lactase deficiency |
| Caused by infection with *Tropheryma whippelii*, a gram-negative rod | Whipple disease |
| Affects the jejunum | Tropical sprue |
| Diagnosed with antigliadin IgG and IgA antibodies, endomysial antibody, antireticulin antibody; and small bowel biopsy shows blunting of intestinal villi | Celiac sprue |
| Periodic acid-Schiff (PAS) + macrophages in intestines | Whipple disease |
| Classic rash of dermatitis herpetiformis | Celiac sprue |
| Causes signs and symptoms of folic acid deficiency including cheilosis, glossitis, stomatitis | Tropical sprue |
| Flatulence after consumption of lactose-containing products | Lactase deficiency |
| Signs and symptoms include hyperpigmentation, arthralgias, rash, diarrhea, endocarditis, ophthalmoplegia, memory deficits, and altered mental status | Whipple disease |
| Avoidance of wheat, rye, and barley will help treat the disorder | Celiac sprue |
| Treated with penicillin | Whipple disease |

# PANCREAS

| | |
|---|---|
| What is pancreatitis? | Inflammation of the pancreas |
| What are the two most common causes of pancreatitis? | 1. Alcoholic pancreatitis<br>2. Gallstone pancreatitis |
| What is the mnemonic for the causes of pancreatitis? | **I GET SMASHED**<br>Idiopathic<br>Gallstones<br>Ethanol<br>Trauma<br>Steroids<br>Mumps<br>Autoimmune<br>Scorpion bites<br>Hyperlipidemia<br>Endoscopic retrograde cholangiopancreatography (ERCP)<br>Drugs (such as thiazide diuretics) |
| What are the signs and symptoms of pancreatitis? | **Epigastric pain that radiates to the back;** nausea, vomiting, decreased bowel sounds, fever |
| What are signs of retroperitoneal bleeding? | **Grey Turner sign and Cullen sign** |
| What is Grey Turner sign? | Ecchymosis seen on the patient flank in hemorrhagic pancreatitis |
| What is Cullen sign? | Periumbilical ecchymosis seen in hemorrhagic pancreatitis |
| What laboratory findings are consistent with pancreatitis? | $\uparrow$ amylase, $\uparrow$ lipase, hypocalcemia |
| What would you expect to see on an abdominal x-ray? | Sentinel loop or colon cutoff sign |
| What is a sentinel loop? | Dilated bowel or air fluid levels near the pancreas |
| What is the colon cutoff sign? | Transverse colon distended with no colonic gas distal to the splenic flexure |

| | |
|---|---|
| **What is the best study to evaluate pancreatitis?** | Abdominal CT |
| **What test should be ordered if there is a suspicion of gallstone pancreatitis?** | Right upper quadrant (RUQ) ultrasound |
| **What is the treatment for pancreatitis?** | Npo, NG tube for ileus or vomiting, IV fluid hydration, and treat the underlying cause |
| **What do we use to determine the prognosis of a patient with pancreatitis?** | Ranson criteria (predicts risk of mortality based on risk factors) |
| **What are Ranson criteria on admission?** | Remember the mnemonic **GA LAW**<br><br>Glucose >200<br>Age >55<br>Lactate dehydrogenase (LDH) >350<br>Aspartate aminotransferase (AST) >250<br>WBC >16,000 |
| **What are Ranson criteria after 48 hours?** | Remember the mnemonic: **C and HOBBS**<br>Calcium <8<br>Hematocrit (Hct) drop >10%<br>Oxygen <60 mm<br>BUN >5<br>Base deficit >4<br>Sequestration of fluid >6 L |
| **How is the risk of mortality calculated based on Ranson criteria?** | <3 risk factors: 1% mortality<br>3-4 risk factors: 16% mortality<br>5-6 risk factors: 40% mortality<br>7-8 risk factors: close to 100% mortality |

# BILIARY TRACT

| | |
|---|---|
| **What is cholelithiasis?** | Gallstones |
| **What are the four classic risk factors for cholelithiasis?** | 1. **Female**<br>2. **Fat**<br>3. **Fertile**<br>4. **Forty** |

| | |
|---|---|
| What is the most common type of stone? | Cholesterol stone |
| What other type of stone can be found? | Pigment stone |
| What is the predisposition to pigment stones? | Hemolytic anemia or hemoglobinopathies |
| Which type of stone is radiopaque? | Pigment stones |
| What are the common signs and symptoms of cholelithiasis? | RUQ pain, nausea, and vomiting especially after a fatty meal |
| What is the most specific and sensitive test to diagnose cholelithiasis? | RUQ ultrasound |
| When should cholelithiasis be treated? | Only if the patient is symptomatic |
| What is the treatment for cholelitihiasis? | Elective cholecystectomy |
| What is cholecystitis? | Gallbladder inflammation secondary to infection caused by an obstructing stone |
| What bacteria cause cholecystitis? | Remember the mnemonic **KEEEP**: *Klebsiella* *E coli* *Enterococcus* *Enterobacter* *Pseudomonas* |
| What are the symptoms of cholecystitis? | **Prolonged RUQ pain, fever,** nausea, vomiting, referred pain to subscapular region on the right + **Murphy's sign** |
| What is Murphy's sign? | Acute pain and inspiratory arrest with deep palpation of RUQ during inspiration |
| How is cholecystitis diagnosed? | RUQ ultrasound, which will show gallstones, gallbladder wall thickening, pericholecystic fluid, and sonographic Murphy's sign |
| What imaging study should be performed if the ultrasound results are equivocal? | Hepatobiliary iminodiacetic acid (HIDA) scan |

What is the treatment for cholecystitis?

Npo, IV fluids, IV antibiotics (third-generation cephalosporin + aminoglycoside + metronidazole, cholecystectomy

What pain medicine has historically been referred to as being more appropriate to treat pain from cholecystitis and why?

Demerol because morphine is thought to cause spasm of the sphincter of Oddi; however, this is not always done in clinical practice

What is choledocholithiasis?

Gallstones in the common bile duct

What are the signs and symptoms of choledocholithiasis/cholangitis?

Jaundice secondary to obstruction, RUQ pain, Murphy's sign, hypercholesterolemia, ↑ alkaline phosphatase, ↑ bilirubin, ↑ alanine aminotransferase (ALT)

What is the treatment for choledocholithiasis?

1. ERCP with papillotomy and stone removal
2. Common bile duct exploration at time of surgery

What are the complications of choledocholithiasis?

Ascending cholangitis and pancreatitis

What is ascending cholangitis?

Bacterial infection of the biliary tract secondary to obstruction

What is the most common organism causing cholangitis?

E coli

What is Courvoisier sign?

Gallbladder enlargement with jaundice secondary to carcinoma of the head of the pancreas leading to a firm palpable gallbladder

What are the classic symptoms of ascending cholangitis?

Charcot triad:

1. Jaundice
2. Fever
3. RUQ tenderness

Or

Reynold's pentad (Charcot triad + altered mental status and shock)

What are the laboratory findings consistent with ascending cholangitis?

↑ WBC, ↑ alkaline phosphatase, ↑ direct bilirubin, ↑ ALT

| | |
|---|---|
| How is ascending cholangitis definitively diagnosed? | ERCP or percutaneous transhepatic cholangiogram (PTC) |
| What is the treatment for ascending cholangitis? | Npo, IV fluids, IV antibiotics (ampicillin + aminoglycoside + metronidazole), and ERCP to remove stones |
| What is primary sclerosing cholangitis? | Chronic inflammation and fibrosis of the biliary tree |
| What is a common medical diagnosis that patients with sclerosing cholangitis also have? | UC |

# LIVER

| | |
|---|---|
| What is cirrhosis? | Chronic hepatic injury leading to fibrosis, necrosis, and nodular regeneration |
| What is the most common cause of cirrhosis? | Alcoholism |
| What are some nonalcoholic causes of cirrhosis? | Alpha-1 antitrypsin deficiency, hemochromatosis, primary or secondary biliary cirrhosis, Wilson disease, hepatitis B, hepatitis C |
| What are the signs and symptoms of cirrhosis? | Jaundice, ascites, asterixis, bleeding, edema, hepatomegaly, encephalopathy, palmar erythema, spider angiomata on the abdomen |
| What is asterixis? | Downward flapping of hands when held in a dorsiflexed position |
| Why do cirrhotic patients get ascites? | Because they have low albumin |
| What is SAAG? | Serum-ascites albumin gradient |
| How is SAAG calculated? | Albumin concentration of serum − albumin concentration of ascites fluid |
| What is SAAG >1.1g/dL indicative of? | Ascites related to portal hypertension |

**What is a SAAG <1.1 g/dL indicative of?**

Non-portal hypertension etiologies of ascites such as nephrotic syndrome, malignancy, tuberculous peritonitis, biliary or pancreatic ascites

**How can the ascites be treated?**

Spironolactone and paracentesis

**What is a major complication of ascites?**

Spontaneous bacterial peritonitis (SBP)

**What is the most common organism causing SBP?**

*E coli*

**What is the most classic sign of SBP?**

Rebound abdominal tenderness in a patient with ascites

**How is SBP diagnosed?**

Paracentesis with fluid sent for cell count and Gram stain, culture, and sensitivity

**What are the diagnostic criteria for SBP?**

Ascites fluid neutrophil count >250 *and* positive Gram stain/culture *OR* ascites fluid neutrophil count >500

**What is the treatment for SBP?**

Third-generation cephalosporin with albumin

**Why do cirrhotic patients tend to bleed?**

PT is elevated and platelets are low.

**What is the treatment for cirrhosis?**

Stop alcohol consumption; multivitamin including thiamine and $B_{12}$; and nutrition

**What marker can detect an alcohol binge?**

Gamma-glutamyltransferase (GGT)

**What is portal hypertension?**

Elevated portal vascular resistance secondary to presinusoidal, postsinusoidal, or sinusoidal obstruction

Presinusoidal: portal vein thrombosis, schistosomiasis

Postsinusoidal: hepatic vein thrombosis, right heart failure

Sinusoidal: cirrhosis

**Internationally, what is the most common cause of portal hypertension?**

Schistosomiasis

What are the classic physical examination findings in a patient with portal hypertension?

Remember the mnemonic **CHASE:**

Caput medusa

Hemorrhoids

Ascites

Splenomegaly

Esophageal varices

What are the treatments for portal hypertension?

Decrease portal pressure with propranolol; transjugular intrahepatic portosystemic shunt (TIPS); last resort is a liver transplant

What is a common cause of hematemesis in a patient with portal hypertension?

Variceal bleeding

How is a variceal bleed diagnosed?

Esophagogastroduodenoscopy (EGD)

What is the treatment for a variceal bleed?

Start with emergent therapy assessing airway, breathing and circulation, initiate IV fluids, if indicated correct clotting factors with fresh frozen plasma (FFP), vitamin K. Vasoactive drugs such as octreotide, somatostatin, or vasopressin have been found to be safer than sclerotherapy to control the bleeding. Sclerotherapy and variceal banding are also options.

Nonselective beta blockers such as propranolol, timolol, and nadolol.

What is the treatment for esophageal varices with no history of bleeding?

If contraindicated—long-acting nitrates

Alternative—variceal ligation

What are some treatments for hepatic encephalopathy?

Lactulose to decrease absorption of ammonia, neomycin, and protein-restricted diet

What is hepatorenal syndrome?

Patients with advanced hepatic disease develop acute renal failure.

How is hepatorenal syndrome diagnosed?

Elevated BUN/creatinine (CR), hyponatremia, oliguria, hypotension, and urine Na <10

What are the three different etiologic categories of hepatitis?

1. Viral (elevated ALT; ALT:AST 2:1)
2. Alcoholic (elevated AST; AST: ALT 2:1)
3. Toxin-induced (Tylenol) (elevated AST)

What is a mnemonic to remember the etiological differences in hepatitis?

virALT

Drugs blAST

Name the hepatitis viruses transmitted via the fecal-oral route.

Hepatitis A and E

Name the hepatitis viruses transmitted via blood and sexual contact.

Hepatitis B, C, D

Name the only DNA hepatic virus.

Hepatitis B

Which hepatitis viruses have a chronic carrier state?

Hepatitis B, C, D

Which hepatitis viruses have a vaccine available?

Hepatitis A and B (and D)

How can you detect an acute hepatitis A infection?

Anti-hepatitis A virus (HAV) IgM

How can you detect immunity to hepatitis A?

Anti-HAV IgG

How is hepatitis A treated?

It is a self-limiting disease.

Which disease state does each of the following hepatitis B markers detect?

HBsAg (hepatitis B surface antigen)  — Active hepatitis or carrier

HBeAg — Chronic hepatitis that is highly infective

HBcAg — Early infection

Anti-HBc IgM — Acute infection (1.5-6 months)

Anti-HBe — Very low infectivity

Anti-HBs — Immune state

Anti-HBc IgG — Remote infection from 6 months to 1 year ago

What can be given to a patient exposed to hepatitis B to prevent infection?

Hepatitis B immunoglobulin (HBIG)

What is the treatment for a person infected with hepatitis B?

Interferon, lamivudine, adefovir

When is the window period for hepatitis B?

The time when HBsAg has become undetectable but HBsAb is not yet detectable (Fig 5-1)

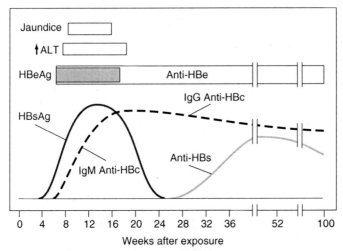

**Figure 5-1** Scheme of typical clinical and laboratory features of acute hepatitis B. *(Reproduced, with permission, from Fauci AS, Braunwald E, Kasper DL.* Harrison's Principles of Internal Medicine. *17th ed. New York: McGraw-Hill; 2008:1934.)*

What is the worst complication of hepatitis B?

Hepatocellular carcinoma

Which hepatitis virus carries the highest risk of developing into hepatocellular carcinoma?

Hepatitis B

What is the treatment for a person infected with hepatitis C?

Interferon + ribavirin

Which hepatitis virus must have concomitant infection with hepatitis B?

Hepatitis D

## CLINICAL VIGNETTES

A 19-year-old male presents to your office complaining of abdominal pain. He describes it as being crampy pain and furthermore he has had diarrhea that is runny in nature. He thinks he has had fever on some occasions as well. You examine the patient and find that this thin male has lower abdominal tenderness with no rebound or guarding. Stool for occult blood is tested and found to be negative. In his mouth you find an aphthous ulcer. What is the most likely diagnosis?

Crohn disease

A 40-year-old obese female presents to the ER complaining of abdominal pain with nausea and vomiting that began 5 hours ago after she ate a large hamburger and French fries. She has had similar symptoms in the past but none that ever lasted this long. Her examination demonstrated the following:

Temp: 101.9°F; BP: 143/85 mm Hg; HR: 80 beats/min; RR: 18; $O_2$ sat: 100%

General: appears to be in pain

Cardiovascular (CV): regular rate and rhythm, no murmurs

Pulmonary: clear bilaterally

Abdomen: soft, tender to palpation in the right upper quadrant; normal bowel sounds

Ext: no clubbing, cyanosis, or edema

What imaging modality would you utilize to try to make the diagnosis?

Ultrasound—It is highly sensitive and specific for detecting cholecystitis.

Your patient complains of midepigastric pain relieve by food for several months. He also complains of nausea and occasional back pain. He is under an immense amount of stress because of the failing economy and all his expenses. A stool *H pylori* comes back positive. What is the appropriate treatment?

Triple therapy: amoxicillin and clarithromycin + bismuth compound + proton pump inhibitor. This patient is also at risk for a duodenal ulcer and should have CBC as well as upper GI endoscopy.

A 35-year-old female comes to the ER complaining of epigastric pain that radiates to the back along with 2 days of nausea, vomiting, and documented fever. The patient admits to drinking two "fifths" of vodka every day. She smells strongly of alcohol. A blood draw demonstrates megaloblastic anemia on CBC, normal kidney function. Liver function tests (LFTs) are elevated also with elevated amylase and lipase. What is the best diagnostic test to make the diagnosis?

Abdominal CT to look for pancreatitis

A 56-year-old male with a history of alcoholism presents to the ER with hematemesis. On examination the patient has a fluid wave, and there are spider angiomata present on his abdomen. He is also clearly jaundiced. His blood pressure is 90/50 with a heart rate of 105 beats/min. You suspect that he has a variceal bleed. What is your first step in treating this patient?

ABCs—Airway establishment, breathing, circulation as well as volume resuscitation with IV fluids

# CHAPTER 6

# Hematology-Oncology

## ANEMIA

What are the three basic categories of anemia?

1. Microcytic (mean corpuscular volume [MCV] <80)
2. Macrocytic (MCV>100)
3. Normocytic (MCV between 80 and 100)

Match the following anemias with their correct category (microcytic, macrocytic, or normocytic):

See Table 6-1.

Iron deficiency anemia

Thalassemia

Folate deficiency

Sideroblastic anemia

Anemia of chronic disease

Lead poisoning

$B_{12}$ deficiency

Chronic renal failure

**Table 6-1** Etiologies of Different Types of Anemia

| Microcytic (Mnemonic: LISTS) | Macrocytic | Normocytic |
|---|---|---|
| Lead poisoning | $B_{12}$ deficiency | Chronic disease |
| Iron deficiency | Folate deficiency | Renal failure |
| Sickle cell anemia | Alcoholism | Aplastic anemia |
| Thalassemias | | Spherocytosis |
| Sideroblastic | | Autoimmune destruction |
| | | Mechanical destruction |

# MICROCYTIC ANEMIAS

**What is the most likely etiology of iron deficiency anemia?**

In women of childbearing age, it is most likely because of menses; in children it is usually a dietary deficiency; and in the elderly it is colon cancer until proven otherwise.

**A 68-year-old man with iron deficiency anemia presents to your clinic and denies any hematochezia or melena. What is the first thing you would do?**

Screen for colon cancer (iron deficiency anemia in the older population is cancer until proven otherwise.)

**What are the symptoms for iron deficiency anemia?**

Pallor, tachycardia, easy fatigability, **Pica, esophageal webs**

**What is the triad for Plummer-Vinson?**

1. Microcytosis
2. Atrophic glossitis
3. Esophageal webs

**What are the laboratory findings seen in iron deficiency anemia?**

↓ iron, ↓ ferritin, ↑ **total iron-binding capacity (TIBC)**, ↓ reticulocyte count

(**Think:** Since there is less iron in the body, there is greater capacity for binding iron.)

**How is iron deficiency anemia treated?**

Ferrous sulfate

**What is sideroblastic anemia?**

Anemia caused by a disorder of the porphyrin pathway leading to ineffective erythropoiesis

**What drugs commonly cause sideroblastic anemia?**

Isoniazid; chloramphenicol, copper chelators, lead

**What are some other causes of sideroblastic anemia?**

Alcoholism, heredity

**What are laboratory findings?**

↑ **Iron,** ↑ ferritin, ↑ **TIBC**

**How is it diagnosed?**

Iron stain of bone marrow shows ringed sideroblasts with Prussian blue stain

**What is the treatment?**

Withdraw the offending agent, if one is identified, and give pyridoxine ($B_6$)

**What type of anemia is sickle cell anemia?**

Microcytic

| | |
|---|---|
| **What kind of genetic inheritance pattern does sickle cell anemia exhibit?** | It is an autosomal recessive disorder |
| **What causes "sickling" of red blood cells (RBCs)?** | Hemoglobin S tetramer polymerizes when RBCs are deoxygenated. |
| **What are some signs and symptoms of sickle cell anemia?** | **Pain crisis** caused by vaso-occlusion<br><br>Infarcts of the lungs, kidneys, bone, spleen<br><br>Intravascular hemolysis<br><br>Osteomyelitis caused by *Salmonella*<br><br>**Aplastic anemia from parvovirus B19 infection**<br><br>Myocardiopathy<br><br>"Fish mouth" vertebrae<br><br>Splenomegaly<br><br>Priapism<br><br>Stroke, transient ischemic attack (TIA) |
| **What kind of infection are sickle cell patients with an autosplenectomy at risk for?** | Infection with **encapsulated bacteria** which include pneumococcus, meningococcus, and *Haemophilus influenzae* |
| **What can intravascular hemolysis lead to in children?** | "Pigment" gallstones |
| **How is sickle cell anemia diagnosed?** | Hemoglobin electrophoresis shows hemoglobin S. |
| **How is sickle cell treated?** | Remember the mnemonic **HOPE:**<br><br>Hydroxyurea—to prevent pain crises<br><br>Oxygen—to prevent sickling of cells<br><br>Pneumococcal vaccine<br><br>Exchange transfusion—when hydroxyurea ineffective |
| **What are thalassemias?** | Hereditary diseases in which there is a decreased production of globins causing a decrease in the production of hemoglobin |
| **What causes alpha-thalassemia?** | A decrease in the alpha-globin chain production. There are four alpha alleles and anywhere from one to all four of these alleles may be affected. |

Match the alpha-thalassemia to the correct number of affected alleles and all the matching characteristics.

See Table 6-2.

| Alpha-thalassemia minor | One affected allele | Hemoglobin Bart ($\beta_4$ hemoglobin) |
| Carrier | Two affected alleles | Mild microcytic anemia |
| Hydrops fetalis | Three affected alleles | Asymptomatic, no anemia |
| Hgb H disease | Four affected alleles | Fetal demise Intraerythrocytic inclusions |

**Table 6-2** Alpha-Thalassemia

|  | Alleles | Characteristics |
| --- | --- | --- |
| Carrier | One allele affected | Asymptomatic |
| Alpha-thalassemia minor | Two alleles affected | Mild microcytic anemia |
| Hgb H disease | Three alleles affected | Intraerythrocytic inclusions |
| Hydrops fetalis | All four alleles affected | Barts; fetal demise |

In what ethnicity is alpha-thalassemia most likely to be found?

More common in Asians. Also seen in people of Mediterranean and African descent.

What causes beta-thalassemia?

A decrease in the synthesis of one or both of the beta chains (there are two beta-chains in hemoglobin.)

In what ethnicities is beta-thalassemia most likely to be found?

African and Mediterranean descent

Match the description below to the correct beta-thalassemia:

| Missing both beta chains | Beta-thalassemia major |
| Missing one beta chain | Beta-thalassemia minor |
| Asymptomatic | Beta-thalassemia minor |
| Splenomegaly, frontal bossing, iron overload | Beta-thalassemia major |
| Treatment is folate supplementation | Beta-thalassemia major |
| Avoid oxidative stress | Beta-thalassemia minor |
| Electrophoresis shows increased fetal hemoglobin (Hgb F) | Beta-thalassemia major |
| Bone marrow transplant | Beta-thalassemia major |

How is beta-thalassemia definitively diagnosed?

Through gel electrophoresis. **Thalassemia major will have increased levels of Hgb F** as well as very decreased Hgb A; while thalassemia minor will have normal levels of Hgb F with somewhat decreased Hgb A.

## MACROCYTIC ANEMIAS

What are five different etiologies of macrocytic anemia?

1. Folate deficiency
2. Vitamin $B_{12}$ deficiency
3. Alcoholism
4. Liver disease
5. Hypothyroidism

Where is vitamin $B_{12}$ absorbed?

In the terminal ileum

What factor is needed for vitamin $B_{12}$ absorption?

Intrinsic factor

What are the signs and symptoms of vitamin $B_{12}$ deficiency?

**Neurologic symptoms** such as ataxia, parasthesias, demyelination of corticospinal tract and dorsal columns. Memory problems can also develop.

What is the most common cause of vitamin $B_{12}$ deficiency?

Pernicious anemia

What is the underlying pathology in pernicious anemia?

In pernicious anemia, there is a decreased production of intrinsic factor because the gastric parietal cells are destroyed by autoantibodies; there is atrophic gastritis.

How is pernicious anemia diagnosed?

↑ Methylmalonic acid

↑ Homocysteine levels

Atrophic gastritis on esophagogastroduodenoscopy (EGD)

**Abnormal Schilling test** (not used as much any more)

What are other causes of vitamin $B_{12}$ deficiency?

Malabsorption because of resection of the terminal ileum or gastric resection, celiac sprue, Crohn disease, infection with *Diphyllobothrium latum* or *Giardia lamblia*. Rarely, $B_{12}$ deficiency is due to hypoalimentation. This can be seen in strict vegetarians or alcoholics.

| | |
|---|---|
| How is vitamin $B_{12}$ deficiency treated? | Vitamin $B_{12}$ supplementation |
| What foods contain folic acid? | Green leafy vegetables |
| Where is folate mainly absorbed? | Jejunum |
| What is the most common cause of folate deficiency? | Hypoalimentation |
| What are other causes of folate deficiency? | Pregnancy, tropical sprue, hemolytic anemia, long-term treatment with bactrim, methotrexate use, 5-flourouricil use |
| What can folate deficiency in pregnancy cause? | Neural tube defects in the developing fetus |
| How can the diagnosis of folate deficiency be differentiated from that of $B_{12}$ deficiency? | **Normal methylmalonic acid** ↑ Homocysteine levels **No neurologic symptoms** |

## NORMOCYTIC ANEMIA

| | |
|---|---|
| What are the most common causes of normocytic anemia? | Anemia of chronic disease, aplastic anemia, renal disease, hemolytic anemia, acute blood loss |
| How is anemia of chronic disease diagnosed? | ↓ Iron; ↓ **TIBC**, normal ferritin |
| Why does renal failure cause anemia? | Erythropoietin is produced by the kidneys, and in chronic renal failure, erythropoietin levels are low. |
| What is the treatment of anemia in a patient with renal failure? | Erythropoietin supplementation |
| What is aplastic anemia? | Bone marrow failure leading to **pancytopenia** |
| Name six different etiologies of aplastic anemia. | 1. Parvovirus B19 in the presence of sickle cell anemia 2. Hepatitis 3. Chloramphenicol 4. Benzene 5. Radiation therapy 6. Idiopathic |

**How is aplastic anemia diagnosed?**

Normocytic, normochromic pancytopenia; hypocellular bone marrow in a bone marrow biopsy

**What are the two main treatments for aplastic anemia?**

1. Bone marrow transplant
2. Immunosuppression

**What is the most common enzyme deficiency that causes hemolytic anemia?**

G6PD deficiency

**Why is G6PD important?**

It is part of the hexose monophosphate pathway which reduces glutathione which is used to protect RBCs against oxidative damage.

**How is G6PD deficiency genetically transferred?**

It is sex-linked.

**In what ethnicities is G6PD deficiency most common?**

Sephardic Jews, Mediterraneans, Middle Easterners, Africans, Asians

**What are the signs and symptoms of G6PD deficiency?**

Signs of hemolysis, which include dark urine, jaundice, weakness, pallor, abdominal and back pain caused by mesenteric/renal ischemia, hepatosplenomegaly.

**What can trigger an attack in a patient with G6PD deficiency?**

Infection, **fava beans**, dapsone, sulfa drugs, primaquine, nonsteroidal anti-inflammatory drugs (NSAIDs)

**What is the pathopneumonic G6PD deficiency diagnostic feature?**

Peripheral smear shows **Heinz bodies, schistocytes, and bite cells.**

**What are Heinz bodies?**

**Inclusions within red blood cells made of denatured hemoglobin**

**What is the treatment for anemia caused by G6PD deficiency?**

It is usually self-limited. Remove inciting factors such as drugs. Transfuse only in very severe cases.

**What two infections are associated with cold autoimmune hemolytic anemia?**

*Mycoplasma* pneumonia and mononucleosis

**Cold autoimmune hemolytic anemia is mediated by which immunoglobulin (Ig)?**

IgM

| | |
|---|---|
| How is cold autoimmune hemolytic anemia diagnosed? | A positive cold agglutinin test or positive indirect Coombs test |
| How is cold autoimmune hemolytic anemia treated? | Staying warm as well as immunosuppresives |
| What general lab results would be seen in hemolytic anemia? | Unconjugated bilirubinemia, hemoglobinuria, elevated urine urobilinogen |

# COAGULOPATHIES

| | |
|---|---|
| What does partial thromboplastin time (PTT) measure? | Intrinsic pathway |
| What does prothrombin time (PT) measure? | Extrinsic and common pathway |
| Which pathway does heparin affect? | Intrinsic pathway |
| Which pathway does warfarin affect? | Extrinsic pathway |
| What are some causes of PT elevation? | Warfarin treatment, vitamin K deficiency, liver disease |
| What are the many causes of thrombocytopenia? | Two categories:<br>1. ↑ Destruction/sequestration<br>Platelet disorders: TTP, ITP, DIC, HUS<br>Splenomegaly<br>Drugs (heparin, aspirin, chemotherapy)<br>2. ↓ Production<br>Leukemia<br>Liver disease/alcohol<br>Aplastic anemia |
| At what platelet level does significant bleeding begin? | 20,000 |
| At what platelet level is a patient at risk for an intercranial bleed? | 10,000 |
| At what platelet level is there an increased risk for bleeding? | ≤50,000 |

Name the platelet disorder associated
with the following features:

Autoimmune-mediated platelet
destruction; often occurs after a viral
infection in children and is self-
limited, can be chronic in adults

ITP (immune thrombocytopenic
purpura)

Triad of thrombocytopenia, hemolytic
anemia, and acute renal failure

HUS (hemolytic uremic syndrome)

Often in children with bloody
diarrhea infected by *Escherichia coli*

HUS

Pentad of fever, anemia,
thrombocytopenia, renal failure,
and neurologic changes

TTP (thrombotic thrombocytopenic
purpura); (Note: **FAT RN**—Fever,
Anemia, Thrombocytopenia, Renal
failure, Neurologic changes)

Seen in adenocarcinoma, trauma,
septic shock, leukemia

DIC (Disseminated intravascular
coagulation)

Often associated with human
immunodeficiency virus (HIV),
malignancy, autoimmune disorders,
pregnancy

TTP

Petechiae and purpura over trunk
and limbs

TTP, ITP, DIC

Caused by the deposition of
abnormal von Willebrand factor
(vWF) multimers

TTP

Describe how each of the following
platelet disorders can be diagnosed:

TTP

Pentad of Fever, Anemia,
Thrombocytopenia, Renal failure,
Neurologic changes in addition to
peripheral smear with **schistocytosis,
helmet cells;** ↓ haptoglobin, ↑ lactate
dehydrogenase (LDH); may have ↑
blood urea nitrogen/creatinine (BUN/
CR), ↑ unconjugated bilirubin

ITP

Diagnosis of exclusion; no fever as in
TTP; no schistocytosis on peripheral
smear; positive Coombs test

DIC

↑ **Fibrin split products,** ↑ **D-dimer,** ↓
fibrinogen, ↑ PT/PTT, ↓ hematocrit

HUS

Stool is hemoccult positive, ↑ BUN/CR,
peripheral smear with schistocytosis,
helmet cells; clinically different from
TTP because there is no change in
mental status

**What is the treatment for each of the following platelet disorders?**

TTP

Plasmapharesis or intravenous immunoglobulin (IVIG) are first-line treatments. Splenectomy in refractory cases. Platelet transfusion is contraindicated because it just causes more consumption of platelets and more symptoms.

ITP

Corticosteroids are first-line treatment; second line is IVIG, splenectomy, or cyclophosphamide

DIC

Treat underlying cause. Platelet transfusion and fresh frozen plasma (FFP) can be given to stop bleeding as first line and aminocaproic acid as second line.

**What is the most common genetic coagulopathy?**

von Willebrand factor deficiency

**How is vWF deficiency inherited?**

Autosomal dominant pattern

**What are the signs and symptoms of vWF deficiency?**

Easy bruisability as well as mucosal and gastrointestinal (GI) bleeding

**How is vWF deficiency diagnosed?**

Normal PT/PTT, ↑ bleeding time, ↓ factor VIII antigen, normal platelet count, ↓ ristocetin platelet study

**What is the treatment for vWF deficiency**

Desmopressin (DDAVP) in mild cases; severe cases need factor VIII concentrate, cryoprecipitate for bleeding

**Name the hemophilia described below:**

X-linked recessive

Hemophilia A

Autosomal recessive

Hemophilia B

Factor IX deficiency

Hemophilia B

Factor VIII deficiency

Hemophilia A

Christmas disease

Hemophilia B

**What are the clinical signs and symptoms of the hemophilias?**

Hemarthroses; bleeding with minimal trauma, multiple ecchymosis

**How are the hemophilias diagnosed?**

↑ PTT, normal PT, normal bleeding time, normal vWF; factor VIII deficiency in hemophilia A and factor IX deficiency in hemophilia B

| | |
|---|---|
| **What is the treatment for each of the hemophilias?** | Hemophilia A: factor VIII concentrate |
| | Hemophilia B: factor IX concentrate |
| **What treatment can be given to a patient with hemophilia A prior to a surgical procedure?** | Desmopressin—It increases the production of endogenous factor VIII |

# LEUKEMIAS

| | |
|---|---|
| **What are the signs and symptoms of leukemia?** | Pallor, fatigue, anemia, infection, petechiae |
| **Name the type of leukemia described below:** | |
| Proliferation of immature blast cells | Acute leukemias |
| Proliferation of mature, differentiated cells | Chronic leukemias |
| Associated with benzene | Acute myelogenous leukemia (AML) |
| Most common leukemia in *children* | Acute lymphoblastic leukemia (ALL) |
| Most common leukemia in *adulthood* | AML |
| Bimodal distribution | Acute leukemias |
| 90% have the Philadelphia chromosome t(9; 22) | Chronic myelogenous leukemia (CML) |
| 30% have the Philadelphia chromosome t(9; 22) | ALL |
| Auer rods, Sudan black positive, myeloperoxidase positive | AML |
| Terminal deoxynucleotidyl transferase (TdT) positive | ALL |
| Blast crisis | CML |
| **What is the peak age of ALL?** | Age 3-4 (most common cancer in children) |
| **What are the subtypes of ALL?** | L1, L2, L3 |
| **What subtype is most common in children?** | 80% are L1. |
| **Of the adult cases of ALL, what subtype is most common?** | L2 |

**What is the L3 subtype morphologically identical?**

Burkitt lymphoma

**How is ALL diagnosed?**

Peripheral blood smear with increased blast cells and **TdT+, periodic acid-Schiff positive (PAS+), CALLA+**

**What is the treatment plan for ALL?**

Induction with chemotherapy (4-5 drugs)

Consolidation

Maintenance—radiation or low-dose chemotherapy

**What is a poor prognostic factor in ALL?**

Presence of Philadelphia chromosome

**What is the treatment in patients who have the presence of the Philadelphia chromosome?**

Bone marrow transplant

**What is the prognosis of ALL in children?**

80% remission

**What is the prognosis in adults?**

30% remission

**What is the most common leukemia in adults?**

AML

**At what age does AML peak?**

Age 15-39

**What are the subtypes of AML?**

M1-M7

M1-M3 granulocyte differentiation

M4-M5 monocytic precursors

M6 erythroblasts

M7 megakaryocytes

**What hematologic disorder is the M3 subtype associated with?**

DIC

**How is AML diagnosed?**

Peripheral blood smear with increased blast cells. Myeloblasts are **myeloperoxidase+, Auer rod+, Sudan black.**

| | |
|---|---|
| What is the treatment for AML? | Induction with daunorubicin and cytarabine; add all-trans retinoic acid for M3 subtype<br><br>Consolidation—continue chemotherapy<br><br>Maintenance |
| What is the prognosis in adults with AML? | Those younger than age 60 have about a 70%-80% remission rate. |
| What age group does chronic lymphocytic leukemia (CLL) affect? | 65 and older |
| Which blood cell type does CLL mainly affect? | B cells |
| How is CLL usually diagnosed? | Bone marrow infiltrated with lymphocytes, lymphocytes express **CD5 protein,** lymphocytosis on complete blood count (CBC) |
| What is the progression of the disease? | Very slow progression |
| What is the treatment for CLL? | Supportive therapy because early therapy does not prolong life. Later there are the COP and CHOP regimens. COP: cyclophosphamide, vincristine, prednisone/prednisolone; CHOP: COP plus doxorubicin. |
| What age group does CML most commonly affect? | 40-60 years of age |
| What carcinogenic agent might CML be associated with? | Prior exposure to radiation |
| What are the unique signs and symptoms of CML? | Abdominal pain/fullness, anorexia, diaphoresis, bone pain |
| What chromosomal abnormality is CML associated with? | 90% have the Philadelphia chromosome. |
| What is the Philadelphia chromosome? | Translocation of the *ABL* gene from chromosome 9 to *BCR* gene on chromosome 22 |

**How is CML diagnosed?**

90% have the Philadelphia chromosome; peripheral blood smear shows increased myeloblasts but less than 30%, basophils, and white blood cells. Low leukocyte alkaline phosphatase.

**What are the different phases of CML?**

1. Chronic phase: hepatosplenomegaly and increase in WBCs
2. Accelerated phase: platelet and RBC decrease while patient develops symptoms of night sweats, fever, bone pain, and weight loss
3. Blastic phase: acute phase of the disease; blood and marrow are rapidly filled with proliferating blast cells

**What is a blast crisis?**

Acute phase of the disease in which the blood and marrow are rapidly filled with proliferating blast cells; this takes about 3-4 years to develop and death is usually within 3-6 months.

**What is the treatment for CML?**

Bone marrow transplant is main treatment. Hydroxyurea and interferon alfa can reduce WBC count. Chemotherapy is for patient who cannot have bone marrow transplant.

**What is the prognosis after a bone marrow transplant in CML?**

About 60% of patients go into remission.

**What can CML progress to?**

AML

**Which type of leukemia has peripheral leukocytes with tartrate-resistant acid phosphatase and cytoplasmic projections?**

Hairy cell leukemia

**What is the treatment for hairy cell leukemia?**

Interferon alfa, splenectomy

# LYMPHOMA

Name the type of lymphoma (Hodgkin lymphoma vs non-Hodgkin lymphoma [NHL]) described below:

Bimodal distribution—peaks in the thirties and seventies, more common in women

Hodgkin lymphoma

Bimodal distribution, more common in men

NHL

Mediastinal lymphadenopathy, contiguous spread

Hodgkin lymphoma

B cells transform to become malignant

Hodgkin lymphoma

Mostly originate from B cells but could also involve T cells

NHL

Peripheral lymphadenopathy, noncontiguous spread

NHL

Associated with Epstein-Barr virus (EBV) infection

NHL—Burkitt lymphoma

Associated with HIV

NHL

Increased pruritus with alcohol consumption

Hodgkin lymphoma

Reed-Sternberg cells

Hodgkin lymphoma

Bone marrow with "starry sky" appearance

NHL—Burkitt lymphoma

What are the four subtypes of Hodgkin lymphoma?

1. Nodular sclerosing
2. Lymphocyte predominating
3. Mixed cellularity
4. Lymphocyte depleted

What is the most common type of Hodgkin lymphoma?

Nodular sclerosing

Which of the four subtypes of Hodgkin lymphoma has the worst prognosis?

Lymphocyte depleted

What clinical feature distinguishes Hodgkin lymphoma from NHL

Adenopathy is regional rather than systemic.

**What are the symptoms of Hodgkin lymphoma and what are they called?**

"B" symptoms—fever, night sweats, malaise, weight loss

**How is Hodgkin lymphoma diagnosed?**

Lymph node biopsy will show Reed-Sternberg cells.

**What are the next steps to be taken after a biopsy determines a lymphoma is present?**

Chest x-ray (CXR) to see extent of involvement as well as possible bone marrow biopsy and computed tomographic (CT) scan

**What is the staging of Hodgkin lymphoma?**

Stage 1: one lymph node

Stage 2: two or more lymph nodes on the same side of the diaphragm

Stage 3: involvement on both sides of the diaphragm

Stage 4: dissemination to organs and tissues

**What is the treatment for Hodgkin lymphoma?**

Radiation therapy for localized disease (stages 1 and 2) and chemotherapy for more extensive disease (stages 3 and 4)

**What chemotherapy regimens are most commonly used?**

ABVD: adriamycin, bleomycin, vincristine, dacarbazine

MOPP: meclorethamine, oncovin, procarbazine, prednisone

**How are the different types of NHL characterized?**

Low, intermediate, and high grade

**Name the most common subtypes of NHL?**

Low grade: follicular small cleaved cell

Intermediate grade: diffuse large-cell lymphoma

High grade: lymphoblastic lymphoma

Burkitt lymphoma: American type and African type

Name the subtype of NHL described
below:

| | |
|---|---|
| High-grade lymphoma more common in children | Burkitt lymphoma |
| Burkitt lymphoma with jaw involvement | African Burkitt lymphoma |
| Burkitt lymphoma with abdominal involvement | American Burkitt |
| Translocation involving *BCL2* gene | Follicular small cleaved cell |
| Can involve the GI tract as well as the head and neck | Diffuse large cell lymphoma |
| Can involve the central nervous system (CNS) and bone marrow | Lymphoblastic lymphoma |
| Derived from thymic T cells | Lymphoblastic lymphoma |

| | |
|---|---|
| How is NHL diagnosed? | Biopsy of lymph node |
| What are the next diagnostic studies to consider after the biopsy? | CXR, CT scan, bone marrow biopsy to determine the extent of the disease |
| What is the prognostic factor in NHL? | Histologic subtype is a more prognostic factor than the extent of spread of disease. |
| How is the adenopathy in NHL described? | Painless adenopathy |
| What is the treatment for NHL? | Radiation and chemotherapy depending on subtype |

# MYELOPROLIFERATIVE DISEASES

| | |
|---|---|
| What are myeloproliferative diseases? | A number of diseases in which there is excessive production of differentiated myeloid cell lines |
| What can the myeloproliferative diseases transform into? | Acute leukemias |
| What is polycythemia vera? | A myeloproliferative disorder in which there is excess production of **ALL** blood cell lines but especially **red blood cells** |

**What are the different etiologies of polycythemia vera?**

It can be a primary disorder which is idiopathic in nature or it can be secondary to hypoxia, dehydration, low erythropoietin production, and smoking.

**What is the peak of onset of polycythemia vera?**

Age >60

**In what sex is polycythemia vera most commonly seen?**

Males

**What are the signs and symptoms of polycythemia vera?**

Pruritis after showering due to basophilia, epistaxis, plethora, blurred vision, splenomegaly, gout, basophilia, headache, retinal hemorrhages, cerebrovascular accidents (CVA), gastric ulcers

**How is polycythemia vera diagnosed?**

On CBC excess of all blood cell lines especially red blood cells. Patient may have low erythropoietin and low erythrocyte sedimentation rate (ESR).

**What is the treatment for polycythemia vera?**

Serial phlebotomy to decrease the volume of blood; hydroxyurea to suppress excess blood cell production; aspirin to thin the blood

**What is a possible long-term complication that occurs in about 20% of patients with polycythemia vera?**

Fibrosis of the bone marrow

**What is essential thrombocytosis?**

Disease in which there is an idiopathic increase of platelets to $>5 \times 10^5$ cells/μL

**What are the clinical signs and symptoms of essential thrombocytosis?**

Burning and throbbing hands and feet as well as splenomegaly; bleeding from nose and gums due to platelet dysfunction

**What are the main treatments for essential thrombocytosis?**

Platelet exchange, hydroxyurea, anagrelide

**What is idiopathic myelofibrosis?**

Disorder in which there is extensive extramedullary hematopoiesis causing replacement of marrow with fibrous connective tissue

| | |
|---|---|
| What is the pathopneumonic sign of myelofibrosis? | Peripheral smear shows **tear drop cells.** |
| What is the treatment for myelofibrosis? | The prognosis is poor and the treatment is mainly supportive. |
| What is multiple myeloma? | Malignant disease of plasma cells which produce **monoclonal immunoglobulins or light chains** |
| What is the ratio of white to African Americans who have multiple myeloma? | 1:2 |
| What can be seen on an x-ray of a patient with multiple myeloma? | Lytic lesions ("punched out" areas of bone) |
| What are the signs and symptoms of multiple myeloma? | Bone pain, pathologic fractures due to **lytic lesions**; anemia, hypercalcemia, renal failure |
| What is the triad that is often seen in multiple myeloma? | 1. Anemia 2. Back pain 3. Renal failure |
| How can multiple myeloma be diagnosed? | 24-hours urine collection followed by urine protein electrophoresis (UPEP) and serum protein electrophoresis (SPEP).These studies will demonstrate free kappa and lambda light chains known as **Bence Jones proteins,** and monoclonal elevation of one cell line. There will be an "M-spike" (or a peak) in the SPEP if there is whole antibody-made. There will be an "M-spike" in the UPEP if light chains only are made. To make the diagnosis there should be a spike in the SPEP or UPEP as well as one of the following: lytic lesions, Bence Jones proteinuria, or increased plasma cells in the bone marrow. |

What is the treatment for multiple myeloma?

Chemotherapy in addition to bisphosphonates and allopurinol as needed for hypercalcemia and elevated uric acid, respectively. Bone Marrow stem cell transplantation is available to some patients. Patients with spinal cord compression are given corticosteroids and/or radiation. Radiation can also be used to treat lesions that are symptomatic.

What is the most common type of plasma cell dyscrasia?

Monoclonal gammopathy of undetermined significance (MGUS)

What is MGUS?

Presence of monoclonal immunoglobulin or M-protein in serum or urine without evidence of any other lymphoproliferative disorder

What are the characteristics that distinguish MGUS from other lymphoproliferative diseases?

Serum M-protein <3 g/dL; no lytic bone lesions, very little or no Bence Jones proteins in urine; bone marrow contains <10% plasma cells, no signs of end-organ damage; patients are asymptomatic

What condition can MGUS patients suddenly develop?

Multiple myeloma

What is the treatment for MGUS?

No treatment is necessary but patients should be followed to make sure they do not develop other lymphoproliferative disorders since these patients are at higher risk.

## CLINICAL VIGNETTES

A 30-year-old male who is known to have atrophic gastritis is found to have anemia on a CBC. His MCV is 105. He also has an elevated methylmalonic acid level and elevated homocysteine level. His vitamin $B_{12}$ level is low. What is the most likely cause of his anemia?

Pernicious anemia

An asymptomatic 50-year-old female is found to have serum M-protein of 4 g/dL. On further examination she is found to have neither Bence Jones proteins on urinalysis nor any evidence of lytic bone lesions on radiographic imaging. Her renal function and liver function tests are within normal limits. What is the most likely diagnosis?

MGUS (monoclonal gammopathy of undetermined significance)

A 20-year-old female presents with a rash on her skin and gingival mucosa. On examination you find that she has petechiae. You also find that she has bruising in many parts of her body. On review of systems she states that she has felt very tired recently. A CBC demonstrated an elevated white blood cell count. A peripheral blood smear was done and showed blast cells as well as Auer rods. What is the diagnosis?

Acute myelogenous leukemia

A 28-year-old female with a past history of HIV is brought in by her brother. He states that she has been acting strangely recently. He states that she seems "confused" recently. He noted a fever as well as petechiae and purpura on her chest. On examination you find hemoglobin of 7 and platelet count of 50,000. Her creatinine is also significantly elevated. What diagnosis do you suspect?

TTP

A 63-year-old male who seems to have a "reddish" complexion presents to your office with complaints of headache and blurred vision. His past medical history is significant for diabetes, stroke, and gastric ulcer. On examination you find him to have a blood pressure of 160/95 and splenomegaly. A CBC demonstrates thrombocytosis. What is this patient's condition called?

Polycythemia vera

# CHAPTER 7

# Rheumatology

## ARTHROPATHIES

| | |
|---|---|
| What is rheumatoid arthritis (RA)? | An autoimmune symmetric inflammatory arthritis |
| What HLA type is RA associated with? | HLA-DR4 |
| In what sex is RA more common? | Females |
| What classical physical examination findings can be found in RA? | Boutonniere deformity; swan neck deformity; ulnar deviation; pain in the **proximal interphalangeal (PIP) and metacarpophalangeal (MCP) joints;** rheumatoid nodules |

What are the seven diagnostic criteria for RA?

1. Morning stiffness >1 hour
2. Three or more joints with arthritis
3. One hand joint with arthritis
4. Symmetric arthritis
5. Rheumatoid nodules
6. Elevated serum rheumatoid factor (RF)
7. Radiographic evidence of erosive arthritis

| | |
|---|---|
| How many of the criteria must be positive for a diagnosis of RA? | Four |
| How long does each of the criteria need to be present to make a diagnosis? | At least 6 weeks |
| What is a boutonniere deformity? | Hyperextension of distal interphalangeal (DIP) and flexion of PIP joints (Fig 7-1) |

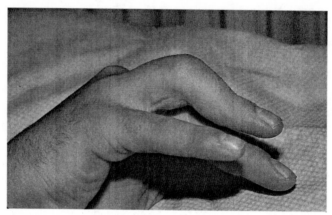

**Figure 7-1**   Boutonniere deformity. (*Reproduced, with permission, from Wilson FC, Lin PP. General Orthopedics. New York: McGraw-Hill; 1997:413.*)

**What is a swan neck deformity?**

Flexion of DIP and extension of PIP joints (Fig 7-2)

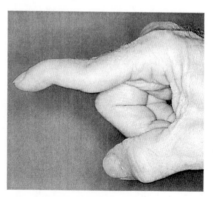

**Figure 7-2**   Swan neck deformity. (*Reproduced, with permission, from Knoop KJ, Stack LB, Storrow AB. Atlas of Emergency Medicine. New York: McGraw-Hill; 1997:291.*)

**What laboratory findings could you expect in a patient with RA?**

↑ RF, ↑ erythrocyte sedimentation rate (ESR)

**What is the treatment for pain associated with RA?**

First-line: nonsteroidal anti-inflammatory drugs (NSAIDs) to decrease inflammation

Second-line: corticosteroids

What disease-modifying agents are available for patients with RA? ✳ | Methotrexate, hydroxychloroquine, gold compounds

What are some newer biologic agents used to treat RA? ✳ | Infliximab, etanercept, abatacept, Rituxan

What is the most common type of arthritis? | Osteoarthritis (OA)

What is the main underlying cause of OA? | Degenerative changes of the joints

What are the two classic physical examination findings in OA? | 1. Heberden nodules which affect the DIP joints
2. Bouchard nodes which affect the PIP joints (Fig 7-3)

*huberdistal*

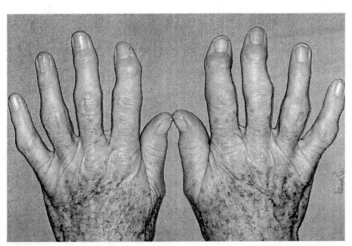

**Figure 7-3**  Bouchard nodes. (*Reproduced, with permission, from Knoop KJ, Stack LB, Storrow AB.* Atlas of Emergency Medicine. *New York: McGraw-Hill; 1997:291.*)

How do the symptoms of OA differ from RA? | Morning stiffness resolves within 30 minutes; outer joints of the hand are mainly affected (DIP joints in addition to MCP and PIP joints).

What are the x-ray findings seen in OA? | Narrowed joint spaces, **osteophyte formation**

What is the treatment for OA? | NSAIDs to relieve pain; muscle-strengthening exercises; steroid joint injection; last resort is joint replacement

| | |
|---|---|
| What is gout? | Arthropathy caused by urate crystal deposit in a single joint |
| What are the etiologies of gout? | Decreased uric acid excretion (high-protein diet, alcohol use, diuretic use) or increased uric acid production (genetic diseases, hemolysis, cancer) |
| What are the signs and symptoms of gout? | Acute pain accompanied by redness and swelling of a joint |
| What is the most common joint to be affected? | First metatarsophalangeal joint |
| What is podagra? | Inflammation of the first metatarsophalangeal joint of the foot which is of sudden onset |
| What are tophi? | Aggregates of gouty crystal and giant cells secondary to chronic gout |
| What is the classic radiographic finding in advanced gout? |  "Rat-bite" appearance |
| How is gout diagnosed? | Fluid aspirated from the joint would reveal **needle**-shaped monosodium urate crystals with **negative birefringence** under polarized light |
| How is acute gout treated? | Colchicine and NSAIDs for pain |
| What is used for maintenance therapy of gout? | Allopurinol to prevent production; probenecid to increase excretion; low-protein diet; refrain from alcohol |
| What is pseudogout? | Deposition of calcium pyrophosphate crystals in joints, causing inflammation |
| What are the risk factors for pseudogout? | Advanced age; gout, hemochromatosis, extensive osteoarthritis, diabetes, hyperparathyroidism, hypothyroidism, hypomagnesemia, neuropathic joint |
| What are the signs and symptoms of pseudogout? | May present as an acute arthritis affecting one or multiple joints like gout, or it may present as a chronic polyarthritis similar to OA or RA |
| What does joint fluid aspiration in pseudogout demonstrate? |  **Positively birefringent** rhomboid crystals |

What is the treatment for pseudogout?    NSAIDs

Name the autoimmune disorder which is characterized by sacroiliitis, with fusion of adjacent vertebral bodies.    Ankylosing spondylitis   → ANT·
WEINS

What HLA type is ankylosing spondylitis associated with?    HLA-B27

What joint is always affected in ankylosing spondylitis?    **Sacroiliac joint**

What are the typical symptoms?    Chronic lower back pain in young men lasting more than 1 hour and relieved with rest

What is the classic x-ray finding seen with ankylosing spondylitis?    **Bamboo spine** (Fig 7-4)

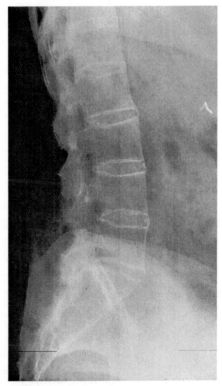

**Figure 7-4**    Bamboo spine. (*Reproduced, with permission, from Wilson FC, Lin PP. General Orthopedics. New York: McGraw-Hill; 1997:454.*)

| | |
|---|---|
| What other disorder is ankylosing spondylitis associated with? | Ulcerative colitis |

## SYSTEMIC DISORDERS

| | |
|---|---|
| What are the signs and symptoms of systemic lupus erythematosus (SLE)? | Fatigue, malaise, malar rash, arthralgias, pericarditis, endocarditis, neurologic symptoms, polyarthritis |
| What is the sex distribution of SLE? | 90% female predominance |
| How is SLE distributed based on race? | Black > white |
| What is the mnemonic for diagnosing SLE? |  DOPAMINE RASH: |

Discoid rash: raised, erythematous circular rash with scale

Oral ulcers

Photosensitivity

Arthritis > 2 joints

Malar rash: butterfly rash on cheeks

Immunologic criteria: anti-Sm Ab, anti–double-stranded DNA, false-positive venereal disease research laboratory (VDRL) test

Neurologic symptoms: seizures, psychosis

ESR elevated (not part of the 11 criteria)

Renal disease

Antinuclear antibody (ANA) positive

Serositis : pericarditis, pleurisy

Hematologic disorder: hemolytic anemia, leukopenia, thrombocytopenia, lymphopenia

| | |
|---|---|
| How many of the criteria must be present to make the diagnosis of SLE? | Four or more |
| What is the pathognomonic heart disorder seen in SLE patients? | **Libman-Sacks endocarditis (LSE)** |
| What autoantibody is most sensitive for SLE? | ANA (it is not specific) |
| Which autoantibody is most specific for SLE? | Anti–double-stranded-DNA (very high titers are associated with renal involvement), anti-SM antibody |

| | |
|---|---|
| What other autoantibodies are associated with SLE? | Anti-La antibody<br>Anti-Ro antibody |
| What are lupus anticoagulant and anticardiolipin associated with? | Thrombosis, central nervous system (CNS) lupus, thrombocytopenia, valvular heart disease, fetal loss |
| What serologies can be falsely positive in patients with SLE? | Rapid plasma reagin (RPR)/VDRL |
| Anticardiolipin can cause a falsely elevated result with which lab test? | Elevated partial thromboplastin time (PTT), but in reality SLE patients are more likely to develop blood clots |
| What are the treatments for SLE? | Avoid sun exposure, NSAIDs for joint pain, systemic steroids, immunosuppressives such as cyclophosphamide in refractory cases with more advanced development of disease |
| How is drug-induced lupus different from SLE? | Symptoms resolve with discontinuation of the drug *and* anti-histone antibody positive |
| What drugs are known to cause drug-induced SLE? | SIQ CHaMP:<br>Sulfasalazine<br>Isoniazid (INH)<br>Quinidine<br>Chlorpromazine<br>Hydralazine<br>a<br>Methyldopa, minocycline<br>Procainamide, penicillamine |
| What is the most common drug to cause lupus-like symptoms? | Procainamide |
| What autoimmune disorder is characterized by systemic fibrosis secondary to excess collagen and extracellular matrix production? | Scleroderma |
| What are the signs and symptoms of scleroderma? | Tight, thick skin; Raynaud phenomenon; dysphagia; renal artery fibrosis; pulmonary hypertension secondary to fibrosis; telangiectasias |

| | |
|---|---|
| What is a more limited form of scleroderma called? | CREST syndrome |
| What does CREST stand for? | Calcinosis<br>Raynaud phenomenon<br>Esophageal dysmotility<br>Sclerodactyly<br>Telangiectasias |
| What laboratory test is 80% sensitive for CREST syndrome? | Anticentromere antibody |
| What laboratory test is highly specific to scleroderma? | Anti–Scl-70 antibody |
| What is the treatment for scleroderma? | Remember the mnemonic CAPS:<br>Calcium channel blocker<br>Ace inhibitor (captopril)<br>Penincillamine<br>Steroids |
| What systemic disease is characterized by noncaseating granulomas in the lung? | Sarcoidosis |
| What race is more predisposed to arcoidosis? | African Americans |
| What are some findings associated with sarcoidosis? | Remember the mnemonic GRUELING:<br>Granulomas<br>RA<br>Uveitis<br>Erythema nodosum<br>Lymphadenopathy<br>Interstitial fibrosis<br>Negative TB test<br>Gamma-globulinemia |
| What renal problem is associated with sarcoidosis? | Nephrolithiasis because of hypercalciuria |
| What is the most important component of diagnosing sarcoidosis? | Transbronchial biopsy showing noncaseating granuloma |
| What is seen on a chest x-ray (CXR) of a patient with sarcoidosis? | Bilateral hilar adenopathy with perihilar calcifications |

What classic laboratory findings are seen in sarcoidosis?

Hypercalcemia and ↑ angiotensin-converting enzyme (ACE)

What is the main treatment for sarcoidosis?

Symptomatic treatment and corticosteroids

What autoimmune disorder is associated with the following triad: keratoconjunctivitis sicca, xerostomia, and arthritis?

Sjögren syndrome

What HLA type is Sjögren syndrome associated with?

HLA-DR3

What type of cancer are patients with Sjögren syndrome at high risk for?

Non-Hodgkin lymphoma

What autoantibodies is Sjögren syndrome associated with?

Anti–single-stranded (SS)-A (Ro) and anti-SS-B (La)

What is the treatment for Sjögren syndrome?

Corticosteroids

Name the syndrome associated with the following: conjunctivitis, uveitis, urethritis, and asymmetric arthritis.

Reiter syndrome

What is the mnemonic used to remember the associated findings of Reiter syndrome?

"Can't see. Can't Pee. Can't climb a tree."
Can't see: conjunctivitis, uveitis
Can't pee : urethritis
Can't climb a tree: arthritis

What HLA type is Reiter syndrome associated with?

HLA-B27

What are the two forms of Reiter syndrome?

1. Sexually transmitted Chlamydia
2. Postinfectious: *Campylobacter, Yersinia, Salmonella, Shigella*

What will a urethral culture often grow out in a patient with Reiter syndrome?

*Chlamydia trachomatis*

What is the treatment for Reiter syndrome?

Doxycycline to cover for *Chlamydia* and NSAIDs for pain

What is the autoimmune syndrome associated with the following: aphthous ulcers, genital ulcers, arthritis, uveitis, psychiatric symptoms

Behçet syndrome

## MUSCLE DISORDERS

What is polymyositis?

Autoimmune disease which causes proximal muscle weakness

How is polymyositis different from dermatomyositis?

Dermatomyositis includes rash as a symptom, whereas with polymyositis there is no rash.

What sex is more likely to have polymyositis?

Females are twice as likely

What are the signs and symptoms of polymyositis?

**Symmetric proximal muscle weakness,** dysphonia, and dysphagia; patients have difficulty standing up from a chair or brushing their hair

What are the classic signs of dermatomyositis?

Symmetric proximal muscle weakness, **heliotropic periorbital rash, shawl sign** (erythematous macules on shoulders and upper back), **Gottron papules** (violacious papules on DIP joints)

What autoantibody is associated with polymyositis and dermatomyositis?

Anti–Jo-1

What are the four criteria for polymyositis?

1. ↑ Creatine phosphokinase (CPK)
2. Proximal muscle weakness
3. Low-amplitude potentials and fibrillations on electromyogram (EMG)
4. ↑ Muscle fiber size on muscle biopsy

What is the treatment for polymyositis and dermatomyositis?

Corticosteroids and methotrexate or cyclophosphamide in refractory cases

What is myasthenia gravis?

Autoimmune disease in which autoantibodies block the postsynaptic acetylcholine receptors preventing acetylcholine from binding leading to muscle weakness

What are the two peak incidences of myasthenia gravis?

Women: second to third decades of life
Men: fifth to sixth decades of life

What can myasthenia gravis be associated with?

Thymomas or other autoimmune diseases

What are the signs and symptoms of myasthenia gravis?

Muscle weakness and increasing fatigue with use, proximal muscle weakness, ptosis, diplopia, dysphagia

What is the "classic" test used to diagnose myasthenia gravis?

Edrophonium test (Tensilon test)

How does the test work?

Edrophonium inhibits acetylcholinesterase allowing for higher levels of acetylcholine to be available to stimulate receptors and, therefore, if the patient has myasthenia gravis, edrophonium administration will lead to improved muscle strength.

What are the newer diagnostic methods for myasthenia gravis?

Single-fiber EMG; anti-acetylcholine receptor antibody test

Myasthenia gravis is often associated with what other finding?

Thymoma

What blood test in the presence of myasthenia gravis is highly associated with the presence of a thymoma?

Anti-striated muscle (SM) antibody—present in >80% of patients younger than 40 with thymoma

What is the treatment for myasthenia gravis?

Pyridostigmine and acetylcholinesterase inhibitor as well as steroids

What is the pathology in Lambert-Eaton syndrome?

There are autoantibodies to presynaptic calcium channels.

How does Lambert-Eaton syndrome differ from myasthenia gravis?

Increased muscle use improves symptoms making muscles stronger.

## VASCULITIS

Name the vasculitis associated with the following:

Small and medium vessel vasculitis with no pulmonary involvement that often presents abdominal pain and is associated with hepatitis B antigenemia and perinuclear antineutrophil cytoplasmic antibodies positive (p-ANCA +)

Polyarteritis nodosa (PAN)

Medium vessel arteritis with prominent pulmonary findings and associated with eosinophilia and asthma

Churg-Strauss disease

Granulomatous vasculitis mainly of the upper and lower respiratory tract that often presents with hemoptysis and can lead to glomerulonephritis

Wegener granulomatosis

| | |
|---|---|
| Cytoplasmic antineutrophil cytoplasmic antibody (c-ANCA) positive | Wegener granulomatosis |
| Medium and large vessel arteritis that is most commonly seen in young Asian individuals | Takayasu arteritis |
| Arteritis that is characterized by loss of pulses in arms and carotids, Raynaud phenomenon, and signs of ischemia such as blindness | Takayasu arteritis |
| Also known as giant cell arteritis and affects the temporal artery | Temporal arteritis |

# CLINICAL VIGNETTES

A 58-year-old male states that the previous evening he had sudden pain and swelling in the great toe of his right foot. Joint fluid aspiration demonstrates negatively birefringent needle-shaped crystals. What is the treatment for an acute attack?

NSAIDs (Colchicine classically)

A 22-year-old male presents with a history of low back pain for the past 6 months. He does not recall any trauma to that area. Rest does not seem to relieve the pain but exercise seems to be helpful. He has decreased range of motion in the lumbar spine. An x-ray demonstrates a "bamboo spine." What is the diagnosis?

Ankylosing spondylitis

A 35-year-old female has photosensitivity, rash on her cheeks, arthritis, and oral ulcers. She also has a positive ANA. You suspect SLE. What serology may be falsely positive in this patient?

RPR/VDRL

A 48-year-old female presents with difficulty swallowing. You notice that her skin appears very shiny, thick, and tight. On review of systems, she mentions that the tips of her fingers become blue and painful in the cold. What laboratory test is specific for the diagnosis of her condition?

Anti–scl-70 antibody to test for scleroderma

An 83-year-old female complains of new-onset headaches. They are unilateral and often unrelieved with NSAIDs. She points to her right temple when asked to describe where the pain is. Her laboratory evaluation demonstrates a significantly elevated ESR. What test would you suggest next to make a diagnosis?

Temporal artery biopsy to evaluate for temporal arteritis

# CHAPTER 8

# Nephrology

## ACUTE RENAL FAILURE

**What is azotemia?**
A high level of urea or other nitrogen-containing compounds in the blood usually secondary to renal failure

**What is acute renal failure (ARF)?**
Newly increased azotemia with an increase in blood urea nitrogen (BUN) and creatinine

**What are the three categories of acute renal failure?**
Prerenal
Renal
Postrenal

**What causes prerenal ARF?**
Low perfusion

**What are examples of prerenal causes of ARF?**
Congestive heart failure (CHF)
Volume loss
Hypotension
Sepsis
Burns
Low blood flow to the kidneys (renal artery stenosis [RAS])

**What is the underlying cause of intrinsic ARF?**
Injury to the nephron due to ischemia or toxins

**What is the most common cause of intrinsic renal failure?**
Acute tubular necrosis (ATN)

**What are some other causes of intrinsic ARF?**
Acute interstitial nephritis (AIN)
Glomerulonephritis (GN)
Ischemia
Vasculitis

What are some causes of postrenal acute renal failure?

Obstruction caused by:

Kidney stones

Enlarged prostate (BPH)

Tumors such as bladder cancer (CA), cervical CA, prostate CA

What are some signs and symptoms of ARF secondary to uremia?

Asterixis, nausea, vomiting, anemia, pericarditis, pruritis, urea crystals on the skin ("uremic frost"), fatigue, oliguria

What are some signs and symptoms of ARF not secondary to uremia?

Metabolic acidosis

Hyperkalemia → arrhythmias

Fluid overload → pulmonary edema, CHF, hypertension

Hyperphosphatemia

Hypertension 2° excess renin secretion

What defines oliguria?

Urine output of <400 cc/24 h

What tests would you initially order to evaluate for ARF?

Urine/serum electrolytes; urine/serum BUN/creatinine (Cr); urinalysis including urine osmolality

What is $FE_{Na}$?

$FE_{Na}$ stands for fractional sodium excretion and is the best diagnostic test to help discriminate between the different types of ARF.

How is $FE_{Na}$ calculated?

$$FE_{Na} = \frac{(\text{urine Na} / \text{plasma Na})}{(\text{urine creatinine} / \text{plasma creatinine})} \times 100\%$$

How do you distinguish between prerenal, renal, and postrenal ARF?

See Table 8-1.

**Table 8-1** ARF: Laboratory Differences Between Prenenal, Renal, and Postrenal Etiologies

| Study | Prerenal | Renal | Postrenal |
|---|---|---|---|
| $FE_{Na}$ | <1% | >2% | >4% |
| Urine Na | <20 | >20 | >40 |
| BUN/Cr | >20 | <15 | >15 |
| Urine osmolality | >500 | <350 | <350 |

Name the type of ARF associated with the following urinary sediment findings:

| | |
|---|---|
| Red cell casts | GN |
| Urine eosinophils | AIN |
| White blood cell (WBC) casts | AIN |
| Granular casts | ATN |

**What are the causes of ATN?**

There are two categories:

1. Ischemic: shock, trauma, hypoxia, hemorrhage, sepsis
2. Toxic: medications, rhabdomyolysis (which causes myoglobinuria), IV contrast

**What medications classically cause ATN?**

Remember the mnemonic **CLAAP:**

Contrast

Lithium

Aminoglycosides

Amphotericin

Pentamine

**How is ATN treated?**

Remove insulting agent, IV fluids to maintain urine output, IV diuretic therapy to increase urinary output and prevent overload, protein-restricted diet, close monitoring of electrolytes; dialysis if needed

**What are the causes of AIN?**

Inflammation of the renal parenchyma caused by:

1. Medications: diuretics, nonsteroidal anti-inflammatory drugs (NSAIDs), penicillin
2. Infection: cytomegalovirus (CMV), Epstein-Barr virus (EBV), toxoplasmosis, syphilis
3. Systemic diseases: Sjögren syndrome, sarcoidosis

**Name the cause of ARF classically indicated by the following serologic tests:**

Anti-neutrophil cytoplasmic antibodies + (ANCA +)

Wegener, polyarteritis nodosa, other vasculitis

Antiglomerular basement membrane antibody (anti-GBM)

Goodpasture syndrome

**How is AIN treated?**

Treatment is the same as ATN.

# CHRONIC RENAL FAILURE

**What is chronic renal failure (CRF)?**

Progressive loss of nephrons

**What is the most common cause of CRF?**

Diabetes

**What is uremia?**

Clinical manifestations of elevated levels of urea in the blood usually secondary to renal failure

**What characterizes uremic syndrome?**

Uremic syndrome is chronic renal failure that has effects on multiple organs and systems.

Cardiovascular: hypertension, pericarditis

Pulmonary: pleural effusions, pulmonary edema

Central nervous system (CNS): asterixis, clonus

Hematology: anemia because of low erythropoietin; increased bleeding time due to platelet dysfunction

Gastrointestinal (GI): nausea; vomiting

Metabolic: acidosis, electrolyte imbalances (especially hyperkalemia), hypocalcemia (lack of vitamin D), azotemia

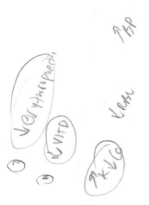

**What can be used to measure the severity of CRF?**

Glomerular filtration rate (GFR); the lower the GFR the worse the renal function

**How is GFR estimated?**

Creatinine clearance is approximately equal to GFR.

| | |
|---|---|
| **How is creatinine clearance calculated?** | Urine creatinine × urine volume in millimeter/serum creatinine × time in minutes |
| | Estimated creatinine clearance = |
| | $$\frac{(140 - age) \times (weight\ in\ kg)\ (for\ females \times 0.85)}{serum\ creatinine \times 72}$$ |
| **In CRF, there is decreased synthesis of what two entities?** | 1. Vitamin D 2. Erythropoietin |
| **What electrolyte abnormalities are seen in CRF?** | Hyperkalemia Hypocalcemia Hyperphosphatemia |
| **What is the treatment for chronic renal failure?** | Dialysis: either hemodialysis or peritoneal dialysis |
| **How should medications prescribed to patients in CRF be adjusted?** | They should be renally dosed. |
| **What are the indications for dialysis?** | Remember the mnemonic **AEIOU:** Acidosis Electrolyte abnormalities Ingestion of toxins Overload of fluid Uremic symptoms |
| **How is vascular access achieved in a hemodialysis patient?** | There are three possible types of access: 1. Arteriovenous (AV) fistula: A shunt between an artery and a vein usually placed in the forearm. Healing may take up to 4 months before it can be used, but once it is healed it may be used for several years. 2. Arteriovenous graft: Often used in patients with small veins that won't properly turn into a fistula. It is a shunt between an artery and a vein using plastic tubing. 3. Catheter: Not permanent. Used until the AV fistula or graft is healed and ready for use. |

| | |
|---|---|
| How is peritoneal dialysis achieved? | Patient gets a permanent catheter in the peritoneum and the peritoneum is used as a membrane through which dialysis is achieved. Dialysis fluid is infused rapidly, then allowed to stay in the peritoneal cavity for several hours, then drained and new fluid infused. |
| What kind of infection are patients on peritoneal dialysis classically at risk for? | Bacterial peritonitis |
| How is bacterial peritonitis treated? | Intraperitoneal vancomycin or antibiotics based on culture sensitivity |

## GLOMERULONEPHROPATHIES

| | |
|---|---|
| What is nephrotic syndrome? | Nephrotic syndrome is glomerular damage leading to proteinuria (>3.5 g/day) |
| What are other defining features of nephrotic syndrome? | Hypoalbuminemia, generalized edema, hyperlipidemia, hypercoagulable state (because of loss of protein C and S), immunocompromised state |
| What is nephritic syndrome? | Glomerular disease leading to syndrome of hematuria, edema, and often hypertension (HTN) |
| How can urinary cholesterol be identified? | If urine is seen under polarized light, there will be "maltese crosses." |
| What are some causes of nephrotic syndrome? | Minimal change disease (MCD) Focal segmental glomerulosclerosis Membranous glomerulonephritis Membranoproliferative glomerulonephritis |
| What are the other names for minimal change disease? | Nil disease, lipoid nephrosis |

Name the nephrotic syndrome associated with each of the following:

| | |
|---|---|
| Loss of epithelial foot processes seen under electron microscopy | Minimal change disease |
| Idiopathic etiology | Minimal change disease |
| Most common primary cause of nephrotic syndrome in adults | Membranous glomerulonephritis |
| Most common primary cause of nephrotic syndrome in children | Minimal change disease |
| Two forms, Type I is slowly progressive and Type II has autoantibodies against C3 and is more rapidly progressive | Membranoproliferative glomerulonephritis |
| Associated with refractory HTN | Focal segmental glomerulosclerosis |
| Frequently recurs | Minimal change disease |
| Granular deposits of IgG and C3 | Membranous glomerulonephritis |
| Often seen in children | Minimal change disease |
| Presents in young, black men with refractory hypertension | Focal segmental glomerulosclerosis |
| Associated with HIV, IV drug abuse, sickle cell anemia | Focal segmental glomerulosclerosis |
| "Spike and dome" on histology due to excess basement membrane | Membranous glomerulonephritis |
| Slowly progressive disease with minimal response to corticosteroid therapy | Membranous glomerulonephritis |
| Does not progress to chronic renal failure | Minimal change disease |
| Associated with hepatitis, systemic lupus erythematosus (SLE), syphilis, malaria, penicillamine, gold salts, CA | Membranous glomerulonephritis |

What is the main treatment for each of the following?

| | |
|---|---|
| Minimal change disease | Corticosteroids |
| Focal segmental glomerulosclerosis | Corticosteroid with cyclophosphamide (prognosis is poor) |
| Membranous glomerulonephritis | Corticosteroids, can add cyclophosphamide in refractory cases |
| Membranoproliferative glomerulonephritis | Corticosteroids. Plasmapharesis can be added. |

Name the systemic diseases that can lead to nephritic syndrome.

SLE, sickle cell anemia, HIV, diabetes, multiple myeloma

What is nephritic syndrome?

Glomerulonephropathy also known as glomerulonephritis in which there is acute-onset hematuria, azotemia, hypertension, edema, and mild proteinuria

What is classically seen on microscopy in nephritic syndrome?

Red blood cell (RBC) casts

Name the five types of glomenrulonephritis.

1. Poststreptococcal glomerulonephritis (PSGN)
2. Rapidly progressive glomerulonephritis
3. Mesangial proliferative glomerulonephritis
4. Membranoproliferative glomerulonephritis
5. IgA nephropathy

Name the nephritic syndrome associated with the following:

Follows group A beta-hemolytic *Streptococcus* or another infectious agent

PSGN

Henoch-Schönlein purpura

IgA nephropathy

Self-limiting disease

PSGN, Henoch-Schönlein purpura

Also known as crescentic glomerulonephritis

Rapidly progressive glomerulonephritis

Goodpasture disease

Rapidly progressive glomerulonephritis

Often diagnosed with elevated ASO titer

PSGN

Buerger disease

IgA nephropathy

Coarse, granular IgG or C3 deposits

PSGN

Smooth, linear IgG deposits

Rapidly progressive glomerulonephritis

Anti-GBM antibody disease

Rapidly progressive glomerulonephritis

What is the most common glomerulonephropathy?

Buerger disease

What is Goodpasture disease?

Glomerulonephritis with pneumonitis

When is the peak incidence of Goodpasture disease?

Males in the second decade of life

What is the most common presenting symptom of Goodpasture disease?

Hemoptysis

## URINARY TRACT

What is nephrolithiasis?

Kidney stones

What are the classic signs and symptoms of nephrolithiasis?

Back pain or flank pain that radiates to groin, nausea, vomiting, microscopic vs gross hematuria

What is the most common type of kidney stone?

Calcium pyrophosphate

What is the underlying etiology?

Hypercalciuria

What is the treatment for calcium pyrophosphate stones?

Hydration and thiazide diuretics; lithotripsy if stone is too large to pass

What is the second most common type of kidney stone?

Ammonium magnesium phosphate

What is another name for ammonium magnesium phosphate stones?

Struvite stones

What are the underlying bacterial etiologies of ammonium magnesium phosphate stones?

*Proteus, Pseudomonas, Providencia,* or *Staphylococcus saprophyticus*

How are struvite stones treated?

Treat the underlying infection and lower the urinary pH

Which type of stone is radiolucent?

Uric acid stones

What disorders are often an underlying cause of uric acid stones?

Gout or myeloproliferative disease

How are uric acid stones treated?

Raise urinary pH

Which type of stone is radiopaque?

Calcium pyrophosphate and ammonium magnesium phosphate

How is nephrolithiasis diagnosed?

Plain films can identify radiopaque stones. Renal ultrasound (US) can visualize hydronephrosis; IV pyelogram is another option. Noncontrast helical computed tomography (CT) scan can visualize small stones and is the gold standard for diagnosis.

What is the most common pathogen in urinary tract infections (UTIs)?

*Escherichia coli*

What is the mnemonic for common pathogens causing UTIs?

**KEEPS:**

*Klebsiella*

*E coli*

*Enterobacter*

*Proteus*

*S saprophyticus*

What are the signs and symptoms of UTI?

Urinary urgency, frequency; burning with urination; hematuria; sense of incomplete bladder emptying

How is a UTI diagnosed?

Urinalysis can demonstrate a high number of WBCs, positive leukocyte esterase, positive nitrites, and moderate to large number of bacteria.

What is the indication of a contaminated urinalysis?

Many epithelial cells or many types of bacteria present

Other than urinalysis, what test should be ordered in a patient suspected to have a UTI?

Urine culture, Gram stain, and sensitivity

What is the first-line treatment for UTI?

3-day course of trimethoprim-sulfamethoxazole (TMP-SMX); however, in areas of high resistance to TMP-SMX, flouroquinalones, typically ciprofloxacin, have become first line

In what type of patient should flouroquinalones be avoided?

Pregnant patients

What would you suspect in a patient with urinary frequency, burning on urination, costovertebral angle tenderness as well as fever and chills?

Pyelonephritis

| | |
|---|---|
| What is the treatment for pyelonephritis? | po or IV antibiotics 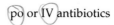 |

## ACID-BASE DISORDERS

| | |
|---|---|
| What are the normal lab values for each of the following components of an arterial blood gas (ABG)? | |
| pH | 7.35-7.45 |
| $Paco_2$ | 35-45 |
| $Pao_2$ | 80-100 |
| $HCO_3$ | 21-27 |
| $O_2$ saturation | 95-100 |
| Base excess | −2 to +2 |
| How is anion gap calculated and what is a normal range? | $Na - (Cl + HCO_3)$. Normal range is 9-14. |
| What is the definition of metabolic acidosis? | ↓ pH with ↓ $HCO_3$ |
| What is Winter's formula? | It determines if there was appropriate compensation in the setting of metabolic acidosis: $1.5 \times (HCO_3^-) + 8 \pm 2 = Pco_2$. |
| What are the causes of anion gap metabolic acidosis? | Remember the mnemonic **MUD PILES:** Methanol, Metformin Uremia DKA (diabetic ketoacidosis) Paraldehyde INH (isoniazid), iron tablets Lactic acidosis Ethanol Salicylates |
| How is the etiology of the metabolic acidosis determined? | Check for ketonuria. |

| Which of the etiologies are present with and without ketonuria? | See Table 8-2. |

**Table 8-2** Anion Gap Metabolic Acidosis Etiologies

| Ketonuria Present | Ketonuria Absent |
|---|---|
| DKA | Lactic acidosis |
| Paraldehyde ingestion | Methanol |
| Isopropyl alcohol ingestion | Ethylene glycol |
| Starvation | Salicylate poisoning |

| What are the causes of normal anion gap metabolic acidosis? | Renal tubular acidosis, diarrhea, colostomy, ileostomy, ingestion of magnesium sulfate, calcium chloride, acetazolamide, hyperparathyroidism |
| What is the treatment for metabolic acidosis? | Correct the underlying cause. |
| What is the definition of respiratory acidosis? | Hypoventilation causing $Paco_2$ and $\downarrow$ pH |
| What is the treatment for respiratory acidosis? | Treat the underlying cause and mechanical hyperventilation can help to release some $CO_2$. |
| What is the definition of metabolic alkalosis? | $\uparrow$ pH, $\uparrow$ plasma bicarbonate, and compensatory $\uparrow$ $Paco_2$ |
| What are the underlying causes of metabolic acidosis? | Vomiting, diarrhea, nasogastric (NG) tube suction for prolonged period, diuretic use, hypomagnesemia, hypokalemia, licorice, tobacco use, Cushing syndrome, RAS |
| What is the treatment for metabolic acidosis? | Treat the underlying cause. These patients are usually volume-depleted so rehydration is needed. Replete potassium and magnesium as needed. |
| What is the definition of respiratory alkalosis? | Hyperventilation causing $\uparrow$ arterial pH, $\downarrow$ $Pco_2$, $\downarrow$ serum bicarbonate |
| What is the treatment of respiratory alkalosis? | Decrease the rate of breathing. |

# RENAL ARTERY STENOSIS

What are the classic findings in renal artery stenosis (RAS)?

Hypertension that is poorly controlled despite multiple medications, often with hypokalemia

What are the underlying causes of RAS?

Atherosclerosis or fibromuscular dysplasia

What is the more common cause of RAS in females?

Fibromuscular dysplasia

What is in the differential diagnosis when a patient has the classic finding of hypertension with hypokalemia?

Conn hyperaldosteronism vs secondary hyperaldosteronism due to renal artery stenosis

How is RAS diagnosed?

Imaging via renal arteriogram, magnetic resonance angiography, or Doppler ultrasonography

How is RAS treated?

Angioplasty and in some cases surgery

# CLINICAL VIGNETTES

Your patient is hospitalized for abdominal pain. During the workup a CT of the abdomen and pelvis is done with contrast. His initial labs showed a slightly elevated WBC count, but otherwise his electrolytes, BUN, creatinine, glucose, AST, ALT, amylase, and lipase were all within normal limits. The following morning, you check the labs and find that the creatinine has suddenly risen dramatically. You check a urinalysis and find that there are granular casts. What class of acute renal failure do you suspect?

Acute tubular necrosis

A 48-year-old male with a past medical history of hypertension and hyperlipidemia rushes to your office. He just had hematuria and he is very concerned. He has also had a very bad sore throat in the last few days. An ASO titer is elevated. What is the most likely reason for this person's hematuria?

Poststreptococcal glomerulonephritis

A 31-year-old female patient comes for follow-up on her hypertension. Despite three different medications, her blood pressure is 148/92. She states that she is very frustrated. She has been trying so hard to follow her low sodium diet, she has been exercising and taking her medications religiously but despite all that her blood pressure is still high. She is also hypokalemic. You suspect renal artery stenosis. What test could be used to definitively diagnose this condition?

Renal angiography

In the patient described in the previous vignette, you find through testing that she does indeed have renal artery stenosis. What is the most likely underlying cause in this particular patient?

Fibromuscular dysplasia

Your patient develops acute renal failure. In your workup you check some labs and calculate a $FE_{Na}$ of 0.5%; urine sodium of 15; urine osmolality above 500. What category of ARF etiologies would you place this patient in?

Prerenal cause

# CHAPTER 9

# Endocrinology

## DIABETES

| | |
|---|---|
| What is the pathophysiology of type 1 diabetes? | Insulin deficiency due to autoinflammatory destruction of pancreatic B cells |
| What is the pathophysiology of type 2 diabetes? | Insulin resistance and relative insulin deficiency |
| What is the age of onset of type 1 and type 2 diabetes? | Type 1 usually begins in childhood/adolescence and type 2 usually begins in adulthood. |
| Which of the two types of diabetes has a stronger genetic factor? | Type 2 diabetes (seems counterintuitive) |
| What are the early symptoms of diabetes? | "The three polys": polyuria, polydipsia, and polyphagia; **and** weight loss |
| What are chronic complications of diabetes? | Retinopathy, nephropathy, neuropathy, cerebrovascular disease, coronary artery disease (CAD), peripheral vascular disease |
| What type of fatal fungal infection can diabetics get? | *Mucor*, especially **sinusitis** (Note: They love to ask this on the boards!) |
| What is the histologic description of *Mucor*? | Nonseptate hyphae with branching at 90° (looks like the letter M) |

**What are the diagnostic criteria for diabetes?**

Both types of diabetes are diagnosed based on the same criteria.

Fasting glucose over 126 two separate times

Random glucose over 200 with symptoms of diabetes

*Or*

Glucose-tolerance test (2-hour test with 75-g glucose load) over 200

**What is the treatment for type 1 diabetes?**

Insulin replacement. Since these individuals do not have insulin, hypoglycemics will not work.

**For each of the following types of insulin, describe the peak and duration of action:**

Lispro (Humalog)

NPH

Glargine (Lantus)

Lente

Levemir

Regular insulin

Ultralente

Aspart (NovoLog)

| Rapid Acting | Peak | Duration |
|---|---|---|
| Lispro | 30-90 min | 3-5 h |
| Aspart | 40-50 min | 3-5h |
| **Short Acting** | | |
| Regular | 2-5 h | 5-8 h |
| **Intermediate Acting** | | |
| NPH | 4-12 h | 18-24 h |
| Lente | 3-10 h | 18-24 h |
| **Long Acting** | | |
| Lantus | No peak | 20-24 h |
| Levemir | 6-8 h | Up to 24 h |
| Ultralente | 10-20 h | 20-36 h |

**Define each of the following complications of insulin treatment:**

Somogyi effect

Nocturnal hypoglycemia causing elevated morning glucose due to release of counterregulatory hormones; treat with less insulin

Dawn phenomenon

Early morning hyperglycemia secondary to nocturnal growth hormone (GH) release

**What is the first-line treatment for type 2 diabetes?**

Metformin

In what patients would metformin be absolutely contraindicated?

In patients who have compromised kidney function because of concern for lactic acidosis

How do we believe metformin works?

Increases sensitivity to insulin

Give an example of each of the following classes of hypoglycemic agents, how they work, and major side effects:

Sulfonylureas

Examples: glipizide, glyburide

(Note: **Start** with GL or end with IDE.)

How they work: increased insulin secretion by B cells

Side effects: hypoglycemia and teratogenic (except glyburide)

Thiazolidinediones

Examples: rosiglitazone (Avandia), pioglitazone (Actose) (end with glitazone).

How they work: increases sensitivity to insulin.

(Note: The **zone** for sensitivity to insulin is increased.)

Side effects: Hepatitis—patients on this class of drugs should have liver enzymes monitored for first year that they are on the drug. Exacerbation of CHF— contraindicated in class III and IV CHF.

When is it most appropriate to treat a type 2 diabetic with insulin?

Refractory to oral hypoglycemic agents

What medication slows the progression of nephropathy in diabetes?

Angiotensin-converting enzyme (ACE) inhibitors and angiotensin receptor blockers (ARBs)

Other than medication, what other therapy is important in diabetes?

Nutrition education

What is HgA1c?

Blood marker of glucose control over the last 3 months. HgA1c <7 is ideal.

What preventative measures are recommended to minimize diabetic complications?

Lipid control (low-density lipoprotein [LDL] <70, TG <150).

BP control <130/80.

HgA1c <7.

Annual foot examinations.

Check for microalbuminuria and proteinuria.

Annual funduscopic examination.

**What is the appropriate treatment in a diabetic patient with microalbuminuria?**

ACE inhibitor or ARB

**What is the major complication of type 1 diabetes?**

Diabetic ketoacidosis (DKA)

**What are the signs and symptoms of DKA?**

Severe hyperglycemia (glucose often >500), ketoacidosis, hyperkalemia, fruity breath, slow deep breaths, abdominal pain, dehydration, lethargy

**What are slow deep breaths in DKA called?**

Kussmaul hyperpnea

**What is the most important treatment in DKA?**

Intravenous (IV) fluid hydration (usually with normal saline)

**What are the other treatments in DKA?**

Insulin drip. Add potassium if potassium is low or normal and add glucose when blood sugar reaches 250 because insulin needs to be continued to be given despite normal glucose until ketones are no longer present.

**What are the most severe complications of DKA treatment?**

Cerebral edema or cardiac arrest due to hyperkalemia

**What is the major complication of type 2 diabetes?**

Hyperosmolar hyperglycemic nonketotic (HHNK) coma; although on rare occasions type 2 diabetics can also go into DKA

**What are some of the signs and symptoms of HHNK?**

Hypovolemia, hyperglycemia (glucose can be >1000), no ketoacidosis, renal failure, altered mental status, seizure, disseminated intravascular coagulation (DIC); often precipitated by acute stress such as trauma or infection.

The difference between HHNK and DKA is that in HHNK there is no ketoacidosis.

**What is the treatment for HHNK?**

The mortality is >50%; as a consequence, immediate treatment is urgent.

Treatment includes rapid IV fluid resuscitation; insulin and potassium are usually needed earlier than in DKA because the intracellular shift of plasma potassium during therapy is accelerated in the absence of acidosis.

# PITUITARY

| | |
|---|---|
| What hormones are secreted from the anterior pituitary? | Follicle-stimulating hormone (FSH), luteinizing hormone (LH), adrenocorticotropic hormone (ACTH), thyroid-stimulating hormone (TSH), prolactin, GH<br><br>(Note: **FAST P:G**) |
| What hormones are secreted from the posterior pituitary? | Vasopressin (antidiuretic hormone), oxytocin |

What is the action of each of the following hormones?

| | |
|---|---|
| FSH | Spermatogenesis in males, ovarian follicle growth in females |
| LH | Testosterone secretion in males and ovulation in females |
| ACTH | Stimulates adrenal cortex to make cortisol, aldosterone, and sex hormones |
| TSH | T3 and T4 production as well as thyroid gland maturation |
| Prolactin | Milk production (lactation) |
| GH | Insulin-like growth factor secretion causing protein and fat metabolism |
| Antidiuretic hormone (ADH), vasopressin | Production of concentrated urine by sodium and water retention |
| Oxytocin | Uterine contractions, milk letdown |

| | |
|---|---|
| What is the most common type of pituitary tumor? | Prolactinoma |
| What type of tumor is a prolactinoma? | A pituitary adenoma which secretes prolactin |
| What are the two mechanisms by which a prolactinoma causes symptoms? | 1. Endocrine effect: due to hyperprolactinemia<br>2. Mass effect: pressure of the tumor on surrounding tissues |
| What are some signs and symptoms of a prolactinoma? | Headache, diplopia, hypogonadism, amenorrhea, gynecomastia, galactorrhea, hypopituitarism |
| What cranial nerve (CN) can be affected by a prolactinoma? | CN III |

| | |
|---|---|
| **How is a prolactinoma diagnosed?** | Magnetic resonance imaging (MRI)/ computed tomography (CT) |
| **What is the first-line treatment for a prolactinoma?** | Dopamine agonist such as bromocriptine |
| **What are other treatment options?** | Surgical resection or radiation therapy if tumor is very large or refractory to medical treatment |
| **Other than a prolactinoma, what are other causes of hypopituitarism?** | Sheehan syndrome (postpartum pituitary necrosis), hemochromatosis, neurosyphilis, tuberculosis (TB), surgical destruction of pituitary |
| **What disorder is seen with elevated levels of GH?** | Acromegaly |
| **What is the most likely underlying cause of acromegaly?** | Pituitary adenoma secreting GH |
| **When must there be an elevation in GH in order for acromegaly to result?** | Elevated levels of GH must be present after epiphyseal closure. |
| **What results if there is excess GH secretion before epiphyseal closure?** | Gigantism |
| **What are the signs and symptoms of acromegaly?** | Coarse facial features, large hands and feet, large jaw, deepening of voice, decreased peripheral vision due to compression of optic chiasm, hyperhidrosis |
| **How is acromegaly diagnosed?** | 1. MRI/CT demonstrating pituitary tumor, 2. Nonsuppressiblity of GH after an oral glucose challenge 3. Elevtated IGF-1 (insulin-like growth factor) |
| **What are the treatment options for acromegaly?** | Surgery or radiation of pituitary tumor, or medical treatment with octreotide or somatostatin, which blocks GH or dopamine agonists |
| **What malignancy are patients with acromegaly at increased risk for?** | Colon cancer |

*(handwritten annotations: "DOPA mine agonist", "tunnel vision", "Somatostatin octreotide", "GH", "IGF-1")*

# THYROID

| | |
|---|---|
| **What is hyperthyroidism?** | Increased secretion of thyroid hormones |
| **In what sex is hyperthyroidism more common?** | Ten times more common in women than men |
| **What is the most common cause of hyperthyroidism?** | Graves disease (80%-90% of US cases) |
| **What are some other causes of hyperthyroidism?** | Plummer disease; toxic multinodular goiter; subacute thyroiditis; amiodarone therapy |
| **What are some of the signs and symptoms of hyperthyroidism?** | **Heat intolerance, weight loss,** exophthalmos, tachycardia, anxiety, palpitations, atrial fibrillation, tremor, sweating, fatigue, weakness, diarrhea, increased reflex amplitude |
| **What is Graves disease?** | Autoimmune disease causing hyperthyroidism. It is due to antibody stimulation of TSH receptors causing excess secretion of free thyroid hormone. |
| **What are the two symptoms only seen in Graves disease?** | 1. Pretibial myxedema 2. Infiltrative ophthalmopathy (exophthalmos) |
| **What is pretibial myxedema?** | Pruritic, nonpitting edema found on shins that usually remits spontaneously |
| **What is infiltrative ophthalmopathy?** | Exophthalmos that may not resolve despite treatment of Graves disease most likely due to autoimmune damage in extraocular muscles |
| **How is Graves disease diagnosed?** | All hyperthyroidism is diagnosed via measurement of TSH, free T4, and free T3. In Graves disease, since there is excess stimulation of the thyroid gland causing increased production of thyroid hormone, laboratory tests show high levels of free T4 and free T3, and low levels of TSH (because of negative feedback) (Table 9-1). Also, a radioactive iodine uptake scan should be done. If uptake is low, then thyroiditis or medication-induced hyperthyroidism is considered. |

**Table 9-1** Thyroid Function Evaluation

| Hyperthyroid | TSH | Free T4 | TRH |
|---|---|---|---|
| Graves disease | ↓ | ↑ | (↑) |
| Pituitary tumor | ↑ | ↑ | ↓ |
| Plummer disease | ↓ | ↑ | (↑) |
| **Hypothyroid** | | | |
| Primary | ↑ | ↓ | ↑ |
| Secondary | ↓ or normal | ↓ | ↑ |
| Tertiary | ↓ or normal | ↓ | ↓ |
| Hashimoto | ↑ | ↓ | ↑ or normal |

TRH, thyrotropin-releasing hormone.

| | |
|---|---|
| **What is another name for toxic multinodular goiter?** | Plummer disease |
| **What is the underlying cause of hyperthyroidism in Plummer disease?** | Multiple thyroid nodules develop autonomous T4 secretion and, therefore, more T4 is released. |
| **How is Plummer disease diagnosed?** | Radioactive iodine uptake tests show "hot" nodules with the rest of the gland being "cold"; also, clinically, nodules can sometimes be felt. |
| **What is another name for subacute thyroiditis?** | de Quervain thyroiditis |
| **What are the signs and symptoms of subacute thyroiditis?** | Prodrome of viral upper respiratory infection (URI) followed by rapid onset of thyroid swelling and **tenderness** as well as hyperthyroid symptoms that can later turn into a hypothyroid state |
| **What is the treatment for de Quervain thyroiditis?** | Usually self-limiting, but aspirin and corticosteroids may be indicated to control inflammation. |

| | |
|---|---|
| What are the treatment options for a hyperthyroid state? | 1. Medication: propylthiouracil (PTU) or methimazole<br>2. Radioactive iodine ablation<br>3. Surgery: subtotal thyroidectomy |
| What is the first-line treatment for Graves disease? | Radioactive iodine ablation except in children and pregnant women |
| What is radioactive iodine ablation? | Radioactive iodine is concentrated in the gland and destroys tissue. |
| What are the possible side effects of radioactive iodine ablation? | Hypothyroidism; thyrotoxic crisis secondary to the release of thyroid hormone into the blood stream |
| What is the mechanism by which PTU works? | It inhibits the peripheral conversion of T4 to T3, decreases iodine uptake, and decreases T4 synthesis. |
| Do patients need to be on therapy for the rest of their lives? | No. After a 1-2 year course of treatment about 50% no longer need to be treated. |
| What are the potential side effects of PTU? | Leukopenia, rash, nausea |
| What other adjunctive treatment is given to patients with hyperthyroidism? | Beta-blocker, usually propranolol, to control symptoms |
| What is the most serious complication of hyperthyroidism? | Thyroid storm |
| What can induce thyroid storm? | Infection, surgery, trauma, abrupt stop of antithyroid medication, serious acute medical problems such as cerebrovascular accident (CVA) or myocardial infarction (MI) |
| What are the signs and symptoms of thyroid storm? | Exaggerated symptoms of hyperthyroidism are tachycardia, high output congestive heart failure (CHF), abdominal pain, hyperpyrexia >104, altered mental status (ultimately coma) |
| What is the mortality rate of thyroid storm? | Up to 50% |

**What is the initial treatment for thyroid storm?**

It is an emergency, so think of the ABCs:

Airway stabilization

Breathing/oxygen administration

Circulation (check pulse/blood pressure [BP]) and start IV fluids

**After primary stabilization of the patient, what is the medical management of thyroid storm?**

The goal of therapy is to decrease circulating thyroid hormone and treat the patient's symptoms.

1. Prevent hormone synthesis: methimazole or PTU
2. Prevent hormone release: cold iodine (about 2 hours after PTU to prevent worsening symptoms)
3. Prevent conversion of T4 to T3: glucocorticoids and beta-blockers
4. Symptomatic treatment: beta-blockers and Tylenol (for fever)

**What are the signs and symptoms of hypothyroidism?**

Cold intolerance, fatigue, lethargy, weakness, **constipation, weight gain,** arthralgias, hoarse voice, skin is dry, coarse, and with nonpitting edema, loss of outer third of eyebrows, delayed relaxation phase of deep tendon reflexes

**What is primary hypothyroidism?**

Thyroid gland dysfunction

**What are some examples of primary hypothyroidism?**

Hashimoto thyroiditis, thyroid ablation or neck radiation therapy in the past, subacute thyroiditis, iodine excess or deficiency, medication-induced

**What medication can cause hypothyroidism?**

Lithium

**What is the most sensitive lab test for primary hypothyroidism?**

Elevated TSH

**What other lab results are present in primary hypothyroidism?**

Low T3 and T4

**What is Hashimoto thyroiditis?**

**Painless** chronic autoimmune thyroid inflammation of autoimmune etiology

**What lab results can help diagnose Hashimoto thyroiditis?**

Elevated antithyroglobulin and antimicrosomal antibody titers

| | |
|---|---|
| What is subacute thyroiditis? | **Tender**, enlarged thyroid; often postviral infection can begin with hyperthyroid symptoms, then hypothyroid symptoms |
| How can you distinguish Hashimoto from subacute thyroiditis? | On clinical examination, in Hashimoto the thyroid gland is **not** tender to palpation but in subacute thyroiditis it is **tender** to palpation. |
| How can Graves disease and Hashimoto thyroiditis be distinguished? | Radioactive iodine uptake is **increased** with Graves and **decreased** with Hashimoto. |
| What is secondary hypothyroidism? | Hypothyroidism caused by pituitary dysfunction |
| What are some examples of secondary hypothyroidism? | Sheehan syndrome, pituitary neoplasm, TB |
| What is Sheehan syndrome? | Postpartum pituitary necrosis |
| What lab results indicate a secondary hypothyroidism? | Low to normal TSH as well as **normal** **thyrotropin-releasing enzyme (TRH)**, low levels of T3 and T4    HIGH (JUST NOT LOW?) |
| What is tertiary hypothyroidism? | Deficiency of TRH |
| What is an example of tertiary hypothyroidism? | Hypothalamic radiation |
| Other than TSH, TRH, T3, T4, what other abnormal lab tests may be found in a hypothyroid patient? | Elevated serum cholesterol (TG, LDL, total cholesterol); elevated aspartate aminotransferase (AST) and alanine aminotransferase (ALT); anemia; hyponatremia |
| What is the treatment for hypothyroidism? | Levothyroxine |
| What is subclinical hypothyroidism? | Elevated TSH levels but with normal thyroid hormone levels and with no clinical symptoms |
| What is the life-threatening complication of hypothyroidism called? | Myxedema coma |
| What are the signs and symptoms of myxedema coma? | Severe lethargy or coma, hypothermia, areflexia, bradycardia |

What causes myxedema coma?

Prolonged cold exposure, infection, sedatives, narcotics, trauma, or surgery

What is the treatment for myxedema coma?

This is an emergency, so start with ABCs (airway, breathing, circulation); IV fluids, steroids, levothyroxine, treat any precipitating causes

What is the initial appropriate workup of a thyroid mass?

Fine-needle biopsy and TSH

What other studies are done to workup a thyroid mass?

Thyroid ultrasound to determine the number and sizes of masses; and thyroid technetium 99m scan

What is a hot nodule and a cold nodule on a thyroid scan?

Hot nodule indicates a hyperactive nodule and is **less** likely to be malignant. A cold nodule indicates a hypoactive nodule that is **more** likely to be malignant.

What is the most common type of thyroid cancer?

Papillary cancer

What is the prognosis for papillary cancer?

85%, 5-year survival

What is seen on pathology?

**Psammoma** bodies, Orphan Annie nucleus

Which type of thyroid carcinoma is associated with multiple endocrine neoplasia types 2 and 3 (MEN 2 and 3)?

Medullary cancer

What can be used to monitor medullary carcinoma?

Calcitonin, because it is a calcitonin-secreting tumor

Which type of thyroid carcinoma has the worst prognosis?

Anaplastic cancer

In what patient population is anaplastic carcinoma usually found?

Older patients

What is the 5-year prognosis for anaplastic carcinoma?

5%-14% survival at 5 years

Which thyroid cancer has the second worst prognosis?

Medullary cancer

| | |
|---|---|
| Which thyroid carcinoma often has metastasis to the bone and lungs? | Follicular cancer  |
| Name the tumors that are part of each of the MEN syndromes. | 1. MEN 1: Wermer syndrome: three Ps: prolactinoma, parathyroid, pancreatoma<br>2. MEN 2: Sipple syndrome: pheochromocytoma, medullary thyroid, parathyroid<br>3. MEN 3: same as MEN 2B: pheochromocytoma, medullary thyroid, mucocutaneous neuromas |

## PARATHYROID

| | |
|---|---|
| What is primary hyperparathyroidism? | Increased secretion of parathyroid hormone (PTH) |
| What is the most common cause of primary hyperparathyroidism? | Adenoma is the most common cause; however, other etiologies include hyperplasia, carcinoma, MEN 2 or 3. |
| What does elevated PTH cause? | There is an ultimate increase in serum calcium (**hypercalcemia**) because PTH leads to increased vitamin D hydroxylation and, therefore, increased calcium resorption as well as decreased resorption of phosphate (**hypophosphatemia**). Calcium levels are also increased because of increased osteoclastic activity (**osteoporosis**). |
| What are the signs and symptoms of hyperparathyroidism? | Same as those for hypercalcemia: **"Stones, moans, groans, and psychiatric overtones."** Because of the osteoclastic activity it can also lead to osteoporosis. |
| What EKG finding could you expect with hyperparathyroidism? | Shortened QT, because of hypercalcemia |
| How is hyperparathyroidism diagnosed? | Hypercalcemia, hypophosphatemia, hypercalciuria, and PTH level |
| What other differential diagnoses should be considered with hypercalcemia? | Neoplasm, sarcoidosis, thiazide diuretic treatment, Paget disease, vitamin D intoxication, milk alkali syndrome, myeloma |

**What is the acute medical treatment for hyperparathyroidism?**

*(handwritten margin note: ZOLEDRONIC ACID, RESIDRONATE, ALENDRONATE)*

Asymptomatic patients with calcium levels below 13 should just be watched. However, symptomatic patients or those with higher calcium levels should be treated with furosemide and bisphosphonates to decrease bone resorption and prevent osteoporosis. Calcitonin can be used as well.

**What long-term treatment must be considered in hyperparathyroidism?**

Surgical treatment. Adenomas should be removed. In hyperplasia, all four parathyroids are removed and a small piece is placed usually near the sternocleidomastoid for functionality.

**What are the most common complications of parathyroidectomy?**

Hoarseness because of damage of the recurrent laryngeal nerve and hypocalcemia

**What is secondary hyperparathyroidism?**

Increased PTH secretion secondary to chronic renal failure or vitamin D deficiency

**What is hypoparathyroidism?**

Decreased PTH

**What are the causes of hypoparathyroidism?**

Idiopathic, DiGeorge syndrome, hypomagnesemia, secondary to surgery or neck irradiation

**Why does hypomagnesemia lead to hypoparathyroidism?**

Because magnesium is necessary for the parathyroid to secrete PTH.

**In what conditions is low magnesium seen?**

Syndrome of inappropriate secretion of antidiuretic hormone (SIADH), pancreatitis, alcoholism

**How is hypoparathyroidism diagnosed?**

Hypocalcemia, hyperphosphatemia, low PTH

**What are the signs and symptoms of hypoparathyroidism?**

Same as that for hypocalcemia: perioral paresthesias, tetany, seizures, Trousseau sign, Chvostek sign, anxiety

**What EKG findings could you expect in hypoparathyroidism?**

Prolonged QT interval because of the hypocalcemia

**What is Trousseau sign?**

Carpal spasm with arterial occlusion with BP cuff

**What is Chvostek sign?**

Spasm of the facial nerve upon tapping

| | |
|---|---|
| How is hypoparathyroidism treated? | Emergently treat with IV calcium, then treat with vitamin D and oral calcium for maintenance treatment. |

## ADRENALS

| | |
|---|---|
| What are the two main parts of the adrenal gland and what is the secretory product of each part? | 1. Adrenal cortex<br>2. Adrenal medulla<br><br>The cortex secretes aldosterone, cortisol, and sex hormones and the medulla secretes the catecholamines including epinephrine and norepinephrine. |
| What is the function of aldosterone? | Kidney resorption of sodium and secretion of potassium and hydrogen ions |
| What is Addison disease? | Primary adrenal insufficiency caused by the destruction of the adrenal cortex leading to a deficiency in both mineralocorticoids as well as glucocorticoids |
| What is secondary adrenal insufficiency? | Decreased secretion of ACTH by the pituitary gland; the adrenal gland is functional |
| What is the cause of tertiary adrenal insufficiency? | Decreased hypothalamic function |
| What is the most likely etiology of Addison disease in the United States? | Autoimmune destruction of the adrenal gland |
| What are some other causes of Addison disease? | TB, amyloidosis, sarcoidosis, HIV, adrenal hemorrhage secondary to DIC or trauma, Waterhouse-Friderichsen syndrome, congenital adrenal hyperplasia, metastasis to the adrenals |
| What is Waterhouse-Friderichsen syndrome? | Endotoxin-mediated adrenal hemorrhage usually caused by meningococcemia that leads to fulminant adrenal failure |
| What is the most likely cause of secondary adrenal insufficiency? | Hypothalamic-pituitary axis disturbance, usually by sudden cessation of exogenous corticosteroids, which leads to decreased ACTH secretion |

**What are some other causes of secondary adrenal insufficiency?**

Pituitary infarction, Sheehan syndrome, pituitary adenoma

**What are some signs and symptoms of Addison disease?**

Because of low aldosterone and cortisol there are hyponatremia, hyperkalemia, pica (craving for salt), weakness, anorexia, hypotension, nausea, vomiting, and hyperpigmentation.

**What are the diagnostic findings in primary adrenal insufficiency?**

Hyperpigmentation, ↑ACTH, ↓ cortisol and aldosterone response to ACTH challenge

**Why do patients get hyperpigmentation?**

ACTH stimulates melanin secretion.

**What is the test used to diagnose adrenal insufficiency?**

ACTH (Cortrosyn) test in which a dose of ACTH is given to the patient and then serum cortisol levels as well as serum ACTH levels are measured about half an hour later

Primary adrenal insufficiency: ↑cortisol levels in response to ACTH and ↑aldosterone levels

Secondary adrenal insufficiency: ↑cortisol levels (more than double normal limits) in response to ACTH and normal aldosterone levels

**How is the diagnosis of secondary adrenal insufficiency distinguished from primary adrenal insufficiency?**

No hyperpigmentation, ↑cortisol response, ↑ACTH

**What kind of metabolic disturbance is seen in primary adrenal insufficiency?**

Metabolic acidosis due to aldosterone and cortisol deficiency and, therefore, lack of secretion of hydrogen ions

**What is the treatment for adrenal insufficiency?**

Glucocorticoid replacement. Extra glucocorticoids should be given in times of physical stress such as infection. You should instruct patients to taper off this extra replacement slowly as to prevent an adrenal crisis.

**What is Cushing syndrome?**

A term used to describe the symptoms caused by hypercortisolism

**How is Cushing *syndrome* different from Cushing *disease*?**

Cushing disease refers to a type of Cushing syndrome caused specifically by ACTH hypersecretion by the pituitary.

| | |
|---|---|
| **What are the different causes of hypercortisolism?** | Exogenous glucocorticoids<br>Pituitary hypersecretion of ACTH<br>Hypersecretion of cortisol due to adrenal hyperplasia/neoplasm<br>Ectopic ACTH production such as with small cell lung carcinoma |
| **What is the most common cause of Cushing syndrome?** | Exogenous corticosteroids |
| **What is the most common cause of endogenous hypercortisolism?** | Cushing **disease** (pituitary hypersecretion of ACTH) |
| **What are the signs and symptoms of Cushing syndrome?** | **Buffalo hump**, moon facies, truncal obesity, striae, virilization/menstrual disorders, hyperglycemia, hypertension, hypokalemia, immune suppression, osteoporosis, hirsutism, acne |
| **What tests are used to diagnose hypercortisolism?** | 24-hour urine-free cortisol and the dexamethasone suppression tests, ACTH level, diurnal cortisol variation |
| **What is the dexamethasone suppression test?** | First a low dose of dexamethasone is given and cortisol is measured. If cortisol is not elevated then Cushing is ruled out; if it is elevated then a high-dose dexamethasone suppression test is done and ACTH is measured. If ACTH is decreased then the pituitary has good feedback and, therefore, it must be an adrenal etiology. However, if the ACTH is high or normal then it is probably ectopic ACTH; and if it is only partially suppressed, then the pituitary is the etiology. Dexamethasone → ↑ACTH (ectopic/pituitary) ↓ACTH (adrenal) |
| **What are some other studies to consider to localize the lesion in hypercortisolism?** | A CT scan can look for an adrenal mass and an MRI can look for a pituitary mass. |
| **What is the treatment for hypercortisolism?** | Treat the underlying cause. If it is a resectable tumor, tumor resection with postoperative glucocorticoids. In nonresectable tumors, medical therapy with ketoconazole, mitotane, metyrapone, or aminoglutethimide. If the etiology is exogenous glucocorticoids; taper off the glucocorticoids and eventually stop. |
| **What is Conn syndrome?** | Primary hyperaldosteronism |

What is the etiology of Conn syndrome?

Either hyperplasia of the zona glomerulosa or aldosterone-producing adenoma

What are the signs and symptoms of Conn syndrome?

Hypertension, muscle cramps, palpitations, polyuria, polydipsia, hypokalemia

What percent of hypertensive patients have Conn syndrome?

1%-2%

What are some of the laboratory findings in Conn syndrome?

↑Na, ↑Cl, ↓K (muscle cramps, palpitations), ↓renin-angiotensin feedback, metabolic alkalosis

What are some ways to diagnose Conn syndrome ?

Captopril stimulation test; fludrocortisone suppression test; sodium loading

What is the captopril stimulation test?

Captopril (an ACE inhibitor) is administered and then serum renin and aldosterone levels are measured. ↑aldosterone and ↓ renin confirm the diagnosis.

What is the fludrocortisone suppression test?

Fludrocortisone, a synthetic corticosteroid, is administered to the patient. Serum aldosterone levels are then measured. In a normal patient it would be expected that aldosterone levels would be suppressed but not in a patient with Conn syndrome.

What is the sodium loading test?

The patient is loaded with sodium via IV saline and then urinary aldosterone levels are tested. No decrease in urinary aldosterone confirms diagnosis.

What is the renin level in Conn syndrome?

Low renin

What other study can help in the diagnosis of Conn syndrome?

CT demonstrating an adrenal nodule or hyperplasia

What is the treatment for Conn syndrome?

Adrenal adenoma: resection of tumor; unilateral adrenal hyperplasia: unilateral adrenalectomy; bilateral adrenal hyperplasia: spironolactone (potassium-sparing diuretic) or ACE inhibitor to control blood pressure

What is secondary hyperaldosteronism?

Elevated aldosterone levels due to elevated renin levels secondary to renal ischemia in CHF, renal artery stenosis, shock, renal tumor.

How is secondary hyperaldosteronism diagnosed?

↓Renin

What can be measured to differentiate primary from secondary hyperaldosteronism?

Renin (this is very important)

What is the treatment for secondary hyperaldosteronism?

Treat the hypertension with a potassium-sparing diuretic, a beta-blocker, and treat the underlying cause.

What is a pheochromocytoma?

Tumor of the adrenal **medulla** that produces excess **catecholamines**

What percentage of people with hypertension have a pheochromocytoma?

0.5%

What are the possible etiologies for a pheochromocytoma?

MEN 2 or 3, von Hippel-Lindau disease, Recklinghausen disease, neurofibromatosis

What are the five Ps of pheochromocytoma?

1. **Pain (headache)**
2. **Pressure**
3. **Perspiration**
4. **Palpitation**
5. **Pallor** and hypertension

What is the most common sign of a pheochromocytoma?

**Hypertension**

What is the diagnostic test for a pheochromocytoma?

Urine screen for elevated **VMA** (vanillylmandelic acid), a urine catecholamine; as well as elevated urine and serum epinephrine and norepinephrine levels

What other test can be done to localize a pheochromocytoma?

A CT scan can identify a **suprarenal mass** (adrenal mass).

What are some other laboratory findings in a pheochromocytoma?

Hyperglycemia, polycythemia

| | |
|---|---|
| What is the "rule of 10s" for a pheochromocytoma? | 10% malignant<br>10% bilateral<br>10% extrarenal<br>10% familial<br>10% in kids<br>10% multiple tumors<br>10% calcified |
| What must be ruled out in a patient with a pheochromocytoma? | MEN type 2 or 3 or |
| What is the treatment for a pheochromocytoma? | In operative cases preoperative alpha-blockers and beta-blockers, then surgical resection; in inoperable cases phenoxybenzámine **or** phentolamine |
| Why treat with preoperative alpha-blockers and beta-blockers? | To prevent unopposed vasoconstriction, and thus volume depletion |

# BONES

| | |
|---|---|
| What is osteoporosis? | Reduction in bone mass leading to increased risk of fracture |
| What are the risk factors for osteoporosis? | Female, postmenopausal or low estrogen state, hypercortisolism, hyperthyroidism, calcium deficiency, low physical activity, smoking |
| What are the typical fractures that occur in osteoporosis? | Hip, vertebrae, and Colle fractures |
| How is osteoporosis diagnosed? | Dual-energy x-ray absorptiometry (DEXA) scan which shows low bone density or an incidental fracture in the elderly |
| What are the treatments for osteoporosis? | Bisphosphonates, calcitonin, selective estrogen receptor modulators, calcium |
| How much calcium should be taken daily? | 1500 mg daily with vitamin D |
| What is the calcitonin most useful for? | Treating bone pain; however, it cannot be used chronically because the effects wear off |

| | |
|---|---|
| What are some examples of selective estrogen modulators? | Tamoxifen, raloxifene |
| What do the selective estrogen modulators increase the risk for? | Thromboembolism |
| What is osteomalacia? | Vitamin D deficiency in adults |
| What is osteomalacia called in children? | Rickets |
| What are the signs and symptoms in children? | **Pigeon breast, craniotabes** (thin skull bones), **rachitic rosary** (costochondral thickening ) |
| How is osteomalacia diagnosed? | Low levels of vitamin D as well as diffuse osteopenia on x-ray |
| How is osteomalacia treated? | Vitamin D supplementation |
| What is Paget disease of the bone? | Localized hyperactivity of the bone which leads to disordered bone matrix being replaced with soft, enlarged bone |
| What is the etiology of Paget? | Unknown, but some think it may be viral |
| What are the signs and symptoms of Paget disease of the bone? | **Hearing loss** (impingement of cranial nerve [CN] VIII), multiple fractures, bone pain, high-output cardiac failure, **increased hat size** |
| What is the typical finding on x-ray? | Hyperlucent area surrounded by hyperdense border-sclerotic lesions |
| How is Paget diagnosed? | **Elevated alkaline phosphatase, sclerotic lesions** on bone scans/x-rays |
| What are the complications associated with Paget disease of the bone? | Pathologic fractures, high-output cardiac failure, hearing loss, kidney stones, sarcoma, spinal cord compression |
| What is the treatment for Paget disease? | Most patients do not need treatment; however, patients with complications associated with Paget disease are treated with bisphosphonates as first line and calcitonin as second line. |

## CLINICAL VIGNETTES

You diagnose a patient with type 2 diabetes. You check a urine microalbumin and find that it is elevated. With what class of medication would you treat this patient?

ACE inhibitor

A 24-year-old male comes to your office complaining of terrible headaches over the past several months. His only past medical history is GERD. He has no past surgical history. The only family history is prostate cancer in his grandfather, otherwise the rest of his family is healthy. On review of systems, he complains of chest palpitations and says that he sweats a lot. His vitals demonstrate a BP of 173/98. On examination you notice that he appears somewhat pale. His cardiovascular, pulmonary, and abdominal examinations are unremarkable. His electrolytes are within normal limits. You suspect a secondary cause of hypertension. What specific diagnostic test would help you screen for your suspected diagnosis?

Urine VMA to screen for pheochromocytoma

Your patient has weight loss, heat intolerance, and palpitations. She complains of swelling and tenderness of her neck. She just got over a head cold. What is the suspected diagnosis?

Subacute thyroiditis

Your diet-controlled diabetic patient presents for a follow-up. The only medication he currently takes is lisinopril. His vitals are as follows: BP: 125/70; P: 73; RR: 15; Temp: afebrile. You review his most recent laboratory tests with him. His HgA1c is 6.8. His urinalysis shows no protein. The lipid profile demonstrates LDL :110, HDL: 45, TG: 100. His most recent fundoscopic examination was 4 months ago and was normal. You do a foot examination and that is normal. What medication change do you suggest?

Add a statin to bring the LDL down below 100.

A 34-year-old male with hypertension presents to your clinic trying to seek your advice regarding his recent weight gain He has gained 20 lb over the course of the last 3 months but denies any change in his diet. He appears to have quite a bit of abdominal girth as well as noticeable striae on his abdomen. His face is also noticeably round and with significant acne. What do you suspect is this patient's condition?

Cushing syndrome

# CHAPTER 10

# Infectious Disease

## HIV/AIDS

| | |
|---|---|
| What is HIV (human immunodeficiency virus? | A retrovirus that destroys CD4 cells |
| How is HIV transmitted? | Sexual contact, blood products, mother to child in HIV positive mothers, needle stick injury |
| How is acquired immunodeficiency syndrome (AIDS) defined? | CD4 count <200 or evidence of an AIDS defining condition or T-helper cell <200/ μL of blood or 14% of all lymphocytes |
| Describe the life cycle of HIV? | gp120 bind CD4 molecule → gp41 molecule helps HIV to fuse with host cell → HIV RNA released into host cell → reverse transcriptase converts viral RNA into DNA → viral DNA translocates into nucleus and viral DNA fuses with host DNA → host cell transcribes the integrated DNA → mRNA is translated into HIV polypeptides which are cleaved by viral proteases → new virus particles assemble to create a new virus cell |
| How is an HIV infection diagnosed? | A positive enzyme-linked immunosorbent assay (ELISA) for HIV is then confirmed with a Western blot assay |
| How is HIV ruled out? | A negative ELISA for HIV |
| What marker is used to follow the *extent* of disease? | CD4 count |
| What can be used as a marker of disease *progression*? | Viral load (it will tell how well the treatment is working) |

| | |
|---|---|
| **What are the signs and symptoms of acute HIV?** | Flu-like symptoms that can later subside |

**Name the complications associated with each of the following CD4 counts:**

| | |
|---|---|
| >500 | Multiple episodes of vaginal candidiasis; lymphadenopathy |
| <400 | Pneumonia, pulmonary TB, oral candidiasis, shingles, Kaposi, non-Hodgkin lymphoma |
| <200 | *Pneumocystis carinii* pneumonia (PCP), wasting, dementia |
| <100 | *Cryptococcus* or toxoplasmosis infections |
| <50 | *Mycobacterium avium* complex (MAC), central nervous system (CNS) lymphoma, cytomegalovirus (CMV), cryptosporidiosis |

| | |
|---|---|
| **When should antiretroviral therapy be initiated?** | At CD4 counts <350 |
| **What is the antiretroviral therapy called?** | Highly active antiretroviral therapy (HAART) |
| **What does HAART therapy usually include?** | Two nucleoside analogues and a protease inhibitor |

**Name the medical management that should be initiated for each of the following CD4 counts:**

| | |
|---|---|
| CD4 <200 | Start prophylaxis against PCP pneumonia and toxoplasmosis with bactrim |
| CD4 <100 | Start prophylaxis against MAC with clarithromycin or azithromycin |
| CD4 <50 | Start prophylaxis against fungal infections with fluconazole |

**Name the AIDS-related opportunistic infection/complication associated with the following:**

| | |
|---|---|
| Presents as nonproductive cough | PCP pneumonia |
| Vascular nodules on the skin | Kaposi sarcoma |
| Most common cause of AIDS death in the United States | Disseminated MAC |
| Most common fungal infections in HIV | Candidiasis |

| | |
|---|---|
| Most common cause of meningitis in AIDS | *Cryptococcus* |
| Presents as painless progressive vision loss | CMV retinitis |
| Painful vesicular eruptions | Shingles |
| Human herpes virus (HHV)-6, 8 | Kaposi sarcoma |
| Bilateral interstitial infiltrates on chest x-ray (CXR) | PCP pneumonia |
| Ring enhancing lesion on head computed tomography (CT) | Toxoplasmosis, CMV, CNS lymphoma |
| Perivascular hemorrhages and exudates on funduscopic examination | CMV |
| Elevated alkaline phosphatase | MAC |

**What is the treatment for each of the following opportunistic infections?**

| | |
|---|---|
| PCP | Bactrim + glucocorticoids |
| Toxoplasmosis | Pyrimethamine + sulfadiazine |
| MAC | Clarithromycin + ethambutol |
| *Cryptococcus* | Amphotericin B + fluconazole |
| CMV | Ganciclovir, foscarnet |
| Shingles | Acyclovir |
| Esophageal candidiasis | Fluconazole, ketoconazole |
| Herpes simplex virus (HSV) | Acyclovir, foscarnet |

# SEXUALLY TRANSMITTED DISEASES

| | |
|---|---|
| Which sexually transmitted disease (STD) is caused by the spirochete *Treponema pallidum*? | Syphilis |

**Name the stage of syphilis associated with the following:**

| | |
|---|---|
| Painless chancre (ulcer) near the area of contact that often heals spontaneously | Primary syphilis |
| Fever, malaise, lymphadenopathy, maculopapular rash on soles and palms, condylomata lata | Secondary syphilis (1-2 months after infection) |

| | |
|---|---|
| Positive serology but asymptomatic and <1 year of infection | Early latent |
| >1 year of infection with possibly positive serology | Late latent |
| Gummas, tabes dorsalis, Argyll Robertson pupil, aortitis, aortic regurgitation, aortic root aneurysm | Tertiary syphilis |

**What are gummas?**

Rubbery granulomatous lesions in CNS, aorta, heart, skin, bone

**What is tabes dorsalis?**

Posterior column degeneration

**How is syphilis diagnosed?**

Four possible tests:

1. Venereal disease research laboratory (VDRL)/rapid plasma reagin (RPR)-rapid test, however nonspecific blood test (eg, can be falsely positive in systemic lupus erythematosus [SLE]).
2. Dark-field microscopy would show motile spirochetes.
3. EIA (enzyme immunoassay): tests for antitreponemal IgG; can be used to screen for syphilis.
4. FTA-ABS/MHA-TP (fluorescent treponemal antibody/ microhemagglutination assay—*T pallidum*): sensitive and specific; it remains positive for life.

**What is the treatment for syphilis?**

Penicillin; doxycycline or tetracycline can be given to penicillin-allergic patients (but not for CNS disease)

**Which STD often coexists with gonorrhea?**

*Chlamydia*

**How can *Chlamydia* present?**

Asymptomatic, cervicitis, urethritis, salpingitis or pelvic inflammatory disease (PID)

**What are the signs and symptoms of *Chlamydia* infection with PID?**

Mucopurulent discharge with adnexal pain

**What is Fitz-Hugh-Curtis syndrome?**

Complication of gonorrhea or *Chlamydia* in which there is perihepatic inflammation and fibrosis

| | |
|---|---|
| What is lymphogranuloma venereum? | Systemic disease caused by the *Chlamydia* L serotype causing painful inguinal lymphadenopathy called buboes |
| What is the treatment for *Chlamydia* infection? | Doxycycline or azithromycin |
| What sexually transmitted disease is caused by a gram-negative diplococcus? | Gonorrhea |
| What is a major complication of gonorrhea? | PID |
| On what type of medium is gonorrhea diagnosed? | Thayer-Martin |
| How is gonorrhea treated? | Third-generation cephalosporin with concomitant treatment of *Chlamydia* |
| How is PID diagnosed? | Cervical motion tenderness plus at least one of the following: positive Gram stain; fever; elevated WBCs, tubo-ovarian abscess; pus on culdocentesis |
| What is the most common cause of vaginitis? | Bacterial vaginosis caused by *Gardnerella* |
| What are the signs and symptoms of vaginitis? | Vaginal itching, burning, bad odor, discharge, and dyspareunia |
| What is the classic odor associated with bacterial vaginosis? | Fishy odor = **positive Whiff test** with KOH prep |
| How is bacterial vaginosis diagnosed? | Clue cells (epithelial cells coated with bacteria) on wet mount |
| How is bacterial vaginosis treated? | Metronidazole |
| Which type of vaginitis is caused by a flagellated, motile protozoan? | *Trichomonas* |
| How is *Trichomonas* diagnosed? | The protozoa are seen on wet mount. |
| What are the classic symptoms of *Trichomonas* infection? | Fishy odor of discharge and **strawberry cervix** |
| How is *Trichomonas* treated? | Patient and partner are treated with metronidazole. |

| | |
|---|---|
| **Which type of vaginitis is associated with a cheesy white discharge?** | *Candida* (also known as yeast infection) |
| **How is candidiasis diagnosed?** | Pseudohyphae on KOH prep |
| **How is a *Candida* infection treated?** | Nystatin cream or oral fluconazole (Diflucan) |
| **Which types of human papillomavirus (HPV) are associated with cervical cancer?** | 16, 18, 31, 45, 51, 52, 53 |
| **What are the two vaccines approved to protect against cervical cancer?** | 1. Gardasil <br> 2. Cervarix |
| **Who should get the vaccine?** | Females aged 12-26 |
| **Which of the two vaccines is also protective against genital warts?** | Gardasil |
| **When should a female start getting Pap smears?** | Age 21 or 3 years after first sexual activity, whichever comes first |
| **How often should a Pap smear be done?** | If a patient has had three normal consecutive Pap smears, they can get them every 3 years after age 30. |

## SEPSIS

| | |
|---|---|
| **What is sepsis?** | An infection that causes systemic inflammatory response syndrome (SIRS) |
| **What is SIRS?** | Includes the following: <br> 1. Tachycardia <br> 2. Tachypnea <br> 3. Fever <br> 4. WBC count >12,000, <4000, or >10% bands |
| **What is septic shock?** | Sepsis-induced hypotension |
| **What type of bacteria causes shock secondary to exotoxin-induced fluid loss?** | Gram-positive bacteria |
| **What type of bacteria causes shock secondary to endotoxin-induced vasodilatation?** | Gram-negative bacteria |

| | |
|---|---|
| What are some of the signs and symptoms of sepsis? | Fever, hypotension, tachycardia, tachypnea, disseminated intravascular coagulation (DIC), increased cardiac output |
| What is the treatment of sepsis? | Intravenous (IV) fluids, antibiotics to treat infection, vasopressors, remove potential sources of infection such as Foley catheter, sometimes steroids |

# OSTEOMYELITIS

| | |
|---|---|
| What is osteomyelitis? | Bone infection |
| What are the two main routes of bone infection? | 1. Direct spread from soft tissue infection<br>2. Hematogenous seeding |
| What types of patients are predisposed to getting osteomyelitis by direct spread? | Diabetics, people with peripheral vascular disease, deep soft tissue injuries |
| What is the most common organism causing osteomyelitis? | *Staphylococcus aureus* |
| What is the most common cause of osteomyelitis in a patient with sickle cell anemia? | *Salmonella* |
| What are the two most common causes of osteomyelitis in a patient who is an IV drug user? | *Pseudomonas, S aureus* |
| What is the most common cause of osteomyelitis in a patient with a deep foot puncture wound? | *Pseudomonas* |
| What are the signs and symptoms of osteomyelitis? | Fever, bone pain, warmth, swelling, erythema of overlying skin, with limited range of motion of the area affected |
| What is the classic finding on x-ray? | Periosteal elevation; lytic lesion |
| What is the gold standard diagnostic technique to evaluate osteomyelitis? | Magnetic resonance imaging (MRI) |
| What is the treatment for osteomyelitis? | Appropriate IV antibiotics for 4-6 weeks |

| What are possible complications of osteomyelitis? | Chronic osteomyelitis, sepsis, septic arthritis, squamous cell carcinoma secondary to a draining sinus tract |
|---|---|

## CLINICAL VIGNETTES

A 32-year-old sexually active female complains of vaginal itching and burning with malodorous discharge. On a wet mount you find epithelial cells coated with bacteria. How do you treat this patient?

Bacterial vaginosis is treated with metronidazole.

Your diabetic patient presents with erythema and swelling over the anterior portion of his shin. It is warm and very painful. He is febrile. He states that his blood sugars have been poorly controlled recently. His HgA1c is 9.6. You get an x-ray and find periosteal elevation. What is the diagnosis?

Osteomyelitis

A 23-year-old sexually active female presents with vaginal discharge. She has also had a fever. A pelvic examination is not tolerated by the patient due to severe pain. You do a Gram stain and find gram-negative diplococci. How do you treat her?

Third-generation cephalosporin to treat the gonorrhea and add doxycycline or azithromycin to cover for a possible coinfection with *Chlamydia*

# CHAPTER 11

# Dermatology

## TERMINOLOGY

Name the primary dermatologic skin lesion described below:

| | |
|---|---|
| Flat, nonpalpable area of discoloration <1 cm in diameter | Macule |
| Elevated, palpable skin lesion <1 cm in diameter | Papule |
| Elevated skin lesion >1 cm in diameter | Plaque |
| | Vesicle |
| Fluid-filled lesion <0.5 cm in diameter | Bullae |
| Fluid-filled lesion >0.5 cm in diameter | Pustule |
| Circumscribed, elevated pus-filled lesion | Wheal |
| Circumscribed, elevated area of edema that occurs transiently | Nodule |
| Circumscribed, elevated solid lesion >0.5 cm | Petechiae |
| Red-purple, nonblanching, pinpoint lesion due to hemorrhage into the skin | Purpura |
| Red-purple, nonblanching lesion >0.5 cm in diameter | Telangiectasia |
| Blanchable lesion due to dilated blood vessel | Lichenification |
| Flat-topped thickening of skin usually due to prolonged scratching | Patch |
| Flat, nonpalpable, >1 cm in diameter | Petechiae |
| Type of lesion seen in any type of thrombocytopenia | |

## SKIN CANCERS

What is the most common type of skin cancer?

Basal cell carcinoma (BCC)

What are the three main characteristic of a BCC seen on physical examination?

1. Pearly papule
2. Telangiectasias
3. Traslucent border

What is the classic description of a BCC?

"Rodent ulcer"(Fig 11-1)

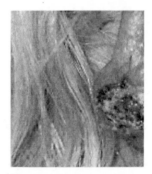

**Figure 11-1** Rodent ulcer. (Courtesy of Noah Craft, MD, PhD)

What is the skin cancer most likely to cause death?

Melanoma

What are the risk factors for BCC (Fig 11-2)?

Sun exposure, fair skin, radiation therapy

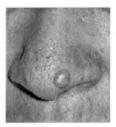

**Figure 11-2** BCC-pearly papule. (Courtesy of Noah Craft, MD, PhD)

Where are BCCs most commonly found?

Sun-exposed skin, ie, head, neck, hands

How is a BCC diagnosed?

Biopsy

What is the treatment?

Excision

What is the prognosis?

Prognosis is excellent because this cancer rarely metastasizes.

What is second most common skin cancer?

Squamous cell carcinoma (SCC)

What is the precursor lesion to SCC?

Actinic keratosis (also known as solar keratosis)

What are the characteristics of an actinic keratosis on physical examination?

Red, scaly, rough patches usually found in sun-exposed area of skin

How are actinic keratoses treated?

Cryotherapy for a small number of lesions, topical 5-FU (an antimitotic agent) for large areas on face and scalp, or imiquimod cream, also photodynamic therapy

What are the risk factors for developing a SCC?

Sun exposure, fair skin, radiation therapy, xeroderma pigmentosa, exposure to arsenic, immunosuppression

Where are SCCs most commonly found?

Sun-exposed areas of skin, ie, head, neck, hand

How is SCC diagnosed?

Biopsy shows "keratin pearls" in the dermis.

What is the treatment?

Excision; radiation in cases where surgery is not an option

What is the prognosis?

Prognosis is very good. They metastasize more often than BCC but not as often as melanoma.

What is the type of skin cancer most likely to be found in younger age groups?

Melanoma (Fig 11-3)

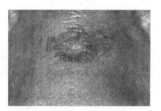

**Figure 11-3**　Melanoma.
(Courtesy of Noah Craft, MD, PhD)

What characteristics are most suggestive of melanoma?

Remember the mnemonic **ABCDEE**:

Asymmetry

Borders are irregular

Colors vary

Diameter is >6 mm (larger than a pencil eraser)

Enlarged over time (growing)

Elevation

What are the risk factors for melanoma?

Sun exposure (particularly childhood sunburn), fair skin, family history

How is melanoma diagnosed?

Excisional or incisional biopsy shows melanocytes with atypia. Do NOT do a shave biopsy.

What is the most important prognostic factor for melanoma?

**Depth** of invasion or thickness of melanoma; the deeper the lesion the worse the prognosis (Fig 11-4)

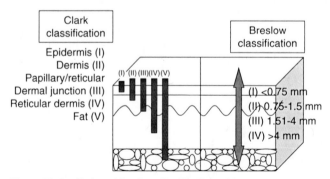

**Figure 11-4**　Clark and Breslow classification schemes.

| | |
|---|---|
| **What is Breslow classification?** | **Breslow classification:** Staging is done by measuring the depth of the lesion in millimeters. |
| **What is Clarke classification?** | **Clarke classification:** Staging is done by determining the penetration of the lesion in relation to the layers of the dermis. |
| **Which classification scheme is most predictive of survival?** | Breslow classification |
| **Name the different types of melanoma.** | 1. Superficial spreading melanoma<br>2. Nodular melanoma<br>3. Lentigo maligna<br>4. Acral lentiginous |

**Name the type of melanoma described below:**

| | |
|---|---|
| **Most common type of melanoma** | Superficial spreading |
| **Melanoma associated with worst prognosis** | Lentigo maligna |
| **Usually found on the head/neck of elderly patient** | Lentigo maligna |
| **Melanoma associated with the best prognosis** | Acral lentiginous |
| **Type of melanoma common in African Americans** | Acral lentiginous |
| **Found on palms, soles, nail beds, mucous membranes** | Form of lentigo maligna that is in radial phase of growth; noninvasive |
| **Hutchinson freckle** | Lentigo Maligna |
| **What is the treatment for melanoma?** | Excision; chemotherapy if metastasis is suspected |
| **What is the type of skin cancer associated with HIV?** | Kaposi sarcoma |
| **Which herpes virus is associated with Kaposi?** | Human herpes virus (HHV) 8 |

What are the clinical findings of Kaposi?

Red/purple macular or papular nodules on skin, mucous membranes, and viscera (especially lungs, gastrointestinal [GI] so it may present as shortness of breath)

What is the treatment?

Treat human immunodeficiency virus (HIV); treat lesions if they cause discomfort; intralesional vinblastine; radiation; chemotherapy

What is mycosis fungoides?

Cutaneous T-cell lymphoma

What is the leukemic phase of the disease called?

Sézary syndrome

What are the clinical findings of mycosis fungoides?

Chronic progressive eczema unresponsive to treatment

## PSORIASIS

What do psoriatic lesions look like?

Pink plaques with silvery-white scale (Fig 11-5)

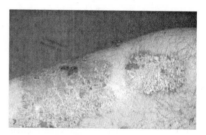

**Figure 11-5**  Psoriasis. (Courtesy of Noah Craft, MD, PhD)

Where are psoriatic plaques classically found?

On the elbows and knees (extensor surfaces)

What other clinical findings can psoriasis be associated with?

1. Fingernail pitting
2. Oncholysis (separation of distal nail plate from nail bed)
3. Psoriatic arthritis (rheumatologic factor negative)

| Which joints do psoriatic arthritis most commonly affect? | Distal interphalangeal (DIP) joints |
| What is Köbner phenomenon? | Psoriatic lesions that occur at the site of injury |
| What is Auspitz sign? | Pinpoint bleeding at sites where overlying scale is removed |
| How is psoriasis affected by season? | Psoriasis is worse in winter and better in summer because sunlight improves lesions. |
| How is psoriasis treated? | See Table 11-1. |

**Table 11-1** Management of Psoriasis

| Topical (Mild Dose) | Systemic (Severe Dose) |
| --- | --- |
| Emollients | Systemic steroids |
| Steroids | Narrow band UV-B |
| Coal tar | Retinoids |
| Vitamin D analogs (calcipotriene) | Methotrexate |
| | Cyclosporine |
| | Biologics |

| What blood tests should be done on patients taking methotrexate? | Complete blood count (CBC) to monitor for bone marrow suppression; liver function test to check for hepatotoxicity; renal function tests |
| What blood test should be done on patients taking cyclosporine? | Renal function tests due to the risk of nephrotoxicity |

## BLISTERING DISEASES

**Name the blistering diseases described below:**

| | |
|---|---|
| Flaccid bullae that rupture easily | Pemphigus vulgaris (PV) |
| Tense bullae that do not rupture easily | Bullous pemphigoid |
| Autoimmune blistering disorder | Both PV and bullous pemphigoid are autoimmune. |
| Blistering disorder more likely to affect 40-60 year olds | PV |
| Blistering disorder most likely to affect the elderly | Bullous pemphigoid |
| Immunofluorescence shows a "tombstone" pattern surrounding epidermal cells | PV |
| Immunofluorescence shows a linear band along the basement membrane | Bullous pemphigoid |
| Blistering disease that is more likely to be fatal | PV (PV is vulgar because it is fatal; that is why we see tombstones on biopsy) |
| Nikolsky sign | Pemphigus vulgaris |

**What is the Nikolsky sign?**

Sloughing of epidermis with gentle traction

**What is the treatment for blistering diseases?**

Oral steroids and antibiotics if infection occurs

## VECTOR-BORNE DISEASES

**Which vector-borne illness is caused by *Rickettsia rickettsii*?**

Rocky Mountain spotted fever (RMSF)

**What are the symptoms?**

Fever, headache, rash, myalgias, nausea, photophobia

(Note: **R**ash **M**yalgias **S**evere headache **F**ever)

**What kind of rash is it?**

Maculopapular

| | |
|---|---|
| **How does the rash spread?** | The rash spreads centrally. It starts at the wrists and ankles and spreads to the palms, soles, and trunk.<br>(Note: The rash **WRAPS: WR**ists **A**nkles **P**alms **S**oles) |
| **In what months is it likely to be seen?** | April through September |
| **In what regions is this illness found?** | It is an illness of the Western hemisphere; mainly southeastern states (North/South Carolina, Tennessee, Oklahoma); rare in the Rocky Mountains |
| **How is RMSF diagnosed?** | Usually a clinical diagnosis with a history of being outdoors or tick bite; clinical test results are slow and it is important to start treatment immediately |
| **What is the most specific and sensitive clinical test for RMSF?** | Indirect fluorescent antibody assay |
| **What are some clinical tests to diagnose RMSF?** | Serologies for *R rickettsii*; Weil-Felix test, biopsy showing necrotizing vasculitis |
| **What is considered the best treatment for RMSF?** | Doxycycline |
| **What is the treatment of RMSF in children?** | Doxycycline, even though tetracyclines are typically not given to children because of the risk of staining teeth, this is one exception. |
| **How would you treat patients that are pregnant but not in the third trimester?** | Chloramphenicol—This is avoided in the third trimester due to the risk of gray baby syndrome. |
| **What is the major side effect of chloramphenicol to watch for?** | Aplastic anemia |
| **What vector-borne illness is caused by *Borrelia burgdorferi*?** | **Lyme disease** |
| **What is this transmitted by?** | Ixodes deer tick |
| **What are the symptoms?** | Fever, headache, myalgias, photophobia, rash, myocarditis |

| | |
|---|---|
| What is the classic rash called and how does it spread? | Erythema chronicum migrans— erythematous annular plaques at the sites of tick bites expand with central clearing<br>(Note: Looks like a target) |
| How is this rash different from that seen in RMSF? | It does not involve the palm and soles; usually rash is on trunk, extremities, axilla, inguinal regions |
| In what months is Lyme disease usually seen? | May through September |
| In what region of the United States is it mostly found? | Northeast |
| How is Lyme disease diagnosed? | Clinically and confirmed by polymerase chain reaction (PCR) or skin biopsy for *B burgdorferi* (spirochete) |
| What is the treatment? | Doxycycline, penicillin |
| What are the potential complications if treatment is delayed? | Cardiac: carditis, atrioventricular (AV) block<br>Neurologic: meningitis, encephalitis, Bell palsy |

# FUNGAL INFECTIONS

| | |
|---|---|
| Name the fungal infection described below: | |
| Scaly, erythematous, pruritic, ring-shaped plaque with elevated borders and central clearing on the body | *Tinea corporis* |
| Previous symptoms found on the scalp | *Tinea capitis* |
| Thickened, yellow fingernails or toenails | *Onychomycosis* |
| Erythematous, scaly plaques with satellite pustules in intertriginous areas | *Candida* |
| Cottagecheese-like plaques on oral mucosa | Oral thrush |
| Sharply demarcated hypopigmented macules on face and trunk; more prominent in summer months | *Tinea versicolor* (also known as *pityriasis versicolor*) |

What is the causative agent of
t versicolor?

*Pityrosporum ovale* also known as
*Malassezia furfur*

How are these infections diagnosed?

KOH (potassium hydroxide)
preparation

What is the "classic finding" on KOH
preparation for *t versicolor*?

**Termed "spaghetti and meatballs"**
(Note: The spaghetti is the hyphae and
the meatballs are the yeast.)

What is seen in the KOH preparation
of *Candida*?

Satellite scrapings show budding yeast
and **pseudohyphae.**

What is seen in KOH preparation of
*t corporis*?

Hyphae

What is the treatment for each of the
following?

T corporis

Topical antifungals (imidazoles)
Systemic antifungals (griseofulvin,
azoles, terbinafine) if unresponsive to
topicals

T versicolor

Topical antifungals; selenium sulfide
shampoo; oral antifungals are rarely
needed

Candida

Reduce moisture and friction in affected
areas usually via weight loss and body
powders; topical antifungals (nystatin)
or oral antifungals

Onychomycosis

**Very difficult to treat!** Oral antifungal
needed

T capitis

Oral antifungal

# BACTERIAL AND VIRAL INFECTIONS

What is the causative agent of acne
vulgaris?

*Propionibacterium acnes* cause
inflammation of the pilosebaceous unit.

What is the term used for a "blackhead?"

Open comedone

What is the term used for a "whitehead?"

Closed comedone

**What are the topical treatments for acne?**

Mild acne: Use topicals alone.

Benzoyl peroxide, retinoic acid, erythromycin, or clindamycin, and antiseptics.

**What are the oral treatments for acne?**

Use in moderate to severe cases (cystic acne).

Oral tetracyclines (doxycycline), erythromycin, clindamycin.

Isotretinoin in very severe cases.

**What is the warning that female patients should receive *before* being placed on an isotretinoin (Accutane)?**

Female patients should be put through the "I Pledge" system and be told that they should **not** become pregnant while taking this drug because it will cause severe fetal abnormalities.

**What is cellulitis?**

Subcutaneous, soft tissue infection with classic signs of inflammation. Area of skin is shiny and poorly demarcated and borders are not elevated.

**What are the classic signs of inflammation?**

**Red** (rubor)

**Hot** (calor)

**Painful** (dolor)

**Swollen** (tumor)

**What are the most common causative agents of cellulitis?**

*Staphylococcus* and *Streptococcus*

**What is the term used to describe a superficial spreading cellulitis?**

Erysipelas

**What is the most common causative agent?**

*Streptococcus pyogenes*

**What patients are at high risk for cellulitis?**

Immunocompromised patients

(Note: If diabetic with tender, erythematous rash on lower extremity unilaterally, **think** cellulitis)

**How is the diagnosis confirmed?**

Gram stain with gram-positive cocci

**How is it treated?**

Penicillin or cephalosporin (cephalexin) If penicillin- or methicillin-resistant *Staphylococcus aureus* (MRSA)-allergic, use vancomycin or clindamycin

| | |
|---|---|
| What are the signs and symptoms of *folliculitis*? | Erythematous pustules in areas of hair growth especially in beard region |
| What is the most common causative agent? | *S aureus* |
| What is the most common causative agent of "hot tub" folliculitis? | *Pseudomonas* |
| What is the treatment? | Keep area clean, if severe can use fluoroquinolone |
| What is a furuncle? | A collection of puss in one hair follicle |
| What is a carbuncle? | A collection of puss in multiple hair follicles |
| What is an abscess? | Localized collection of pus "walled off" by a cavity formed by the surrounding tissue |
| What is the most common causative agent? | *S aureus* |
| What is the abnormal lab value seen? | High white blood cell (WBC) count |
| What is the treatment for an abscess, carbuncle, and furuncle? | Incision and drainage; antibiotics may be added if needed (cephalexin is typical but it does not cover MRSA which has become more prevalent and may need an antibiotic such as clindamycin or Bactrim ) |
| What is impetigo? | Superficial skin infection |
| What is the characteristic description of impetigo? | **Honey-crusted lesion** |
| What is the treatment? | Cephalexin, clindamycin (if MRSA) |
| What are the most common causative agents? | *S aureus* (children) or *S pyogenes* (adults) |
| What is erythrasma? | An **eryth**ematous rash along major skin folds (eg, axilla, groin) |
| In what patient population is it most commonly found? | Diabetics |

| | |
|---|---|
| **What is the causative agent?** | *Corynebacterium* |
| **How is it diagnosed?** | Under Wood lamp there is coral red fluorescence; KOH preparation is negative. |
| **What is the treatment?** | Erythrasma is treated with erythromycin. |
| **What is the term used to describe a plugged apocrine sweat gland that has become infected?** | Hidradenitis suppurativa |
| **In what regions of the body is it usually found?** | Axilla and groin |
| **What is the treatment?** | Surgical debridement and antibiotics |
| **What is the term used to describe an infection of the skin surrounding the nail plate?** | Paronychia |
| **What are the most common infective agents?** | *Staphylococcus or Streptococcus* |
| **What is the treatment?** | Warm compress, incision and drainage (ID) if purulent, keflex if severe |
| **What is herpes simplex?** | Recurrent, painful vesicular eruptions in groups due to the herpes simplex virus (HSV) infection |
| **Where are the lesions most commonly found?** | Oral-labial region or genitals |
| **What form of the virus is most commonly found at each of the regions above?** | HSV 1: oral-labial HSV 2: genital (Note: **Think from top to bottom—type 1 then type 2) (Fig 11-6)** |

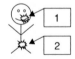

**Figure 11-6** Typical locations of HSV 1 and HSV 2 eruptions.

**How is it diagnosed?**

**Tzanck smear**—positive for HSV when multinucleated giant cells are seen

**What is the treatment?**

Acyclovir ointment reduces duration but does not prevent recurrence. Oral acyclovir reduces frequency and recurrence.

**What is herpes zoster?**

Also known as shingles; an acute, dermatomal vesicular eruption caused by the reactivation of latent varicella zoster that has been dormant in the sensory root ganglion (Fig 11-7)

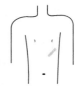

**Figure 11-7**    Dermatomal distribution of herpes zoster.

**What is the typical history of symptoms?**

Day 1: dermatomal pain (no lesions), can also present with fever, malaise

Day 3-5: **unilateral** grouped vesicles along a dermatome

Day 5-10: crust formation

**Which nerves are most commonly involved?**

Thoracic nerves

**What test is used to confirm the diagnosis?**

Tzanck smear—multinucleated giant cells revealed (same as with herpes simplex)

**What is the term used to describe herpes infection of the geniculate ganglion which leads to vesicles forming on the external auditory meatus?**

Ramsay Hunt syndrome (RHS)

**What can happen if RHS is not treated rapidly?**

It could extend to meningitis. It can also lead to facial paralysis and hearing loss.

**What is the treatment for herpes zoster?**

Oral acyclovir within 3 days of infection; immunocompromised patient: IV acyclovir

Analgesia to all patients (**it hurts**)

| What are potential complications of herpes zoster? | 1. Superficial infection of affected area.<br>2. **Postherpetic neuralgia** (may last for years).<br>3. V1 (primary visual area) involvement can lead to corneal scarring. |

## PIGMENTARY DISORDERS

Name the pigmentary disorders described below:

| Discrete areas of hypopigmentation due to melanocyte loss | Vitiligo |
| Hypopigmentation due to tyrosinase deficiency—melanocytes present | Albinism |
| Dark hyperpigmented plaques on flexor surfaces and intertriginous areas | Acanthosis nigricans |

| What autoimmune disorder is associated with vitiligo? | Thyroid disease |
| What are the potential treatments for vitiligo? | Vitiligo cannot be cured because it is autoimmune in nature, but skin grafting or total depigmentation are options, also psoralen–UV-A (PUVA) and narrow band UV-B |
| What are the characteristics seen in albinism? | White skin and hair, red eyes, translucent iris, impaired vision with nystagmus |
| What are albinos predisposed to? | Skin cancer |
| In what patient population is acanthosis nigricans seen? | Obese patients and patients with diabetes |
| What can acanthosis nigricans be a sign of? | It may indicate the presence of a malignancy. |

# HYPERSENSITIVITY REACTIONS

What is Henoch-Schönlein purpura?

An IgA small vessel hypersensitivity vasculitis in which immune complexes lodge in small vessels resulting in inflammation, fibrinoid necrosis, and **palpable purpura**. Patients have a hypersensitivity reaction to antigens in immune complex.

What is seen on physical examination?

**Palpable purpura,** usually of the lower extremities and buttocks.

Lesions may be crusted because of tissue necrosis.

Patients also present with abdominal pain, pruritis, fever, and malaise.

What is palpable purpura?

Nonblanchable, red papules

What patient population is Henoch-Schönlein purpura usually seen in?

Children

What are the criteria for diagnosis of a hypersensitivity vasculitis according to the American College of Rheumatology?

Three of the following must be present:

Meds taken at onset of disease

Age >16 at onset of disease

Palpable purpura

Maculopapular rash

Eosinophils seen on biopsy

What can it potentially progress to and why?

Rarely it progresses to glomerulonephritis because IgA deposits in glomeruli.

What is the treatment?

Treat the underlying cause; systemic corticosteroids; immunosuppressives in serious cases but often self-limiting

What is erythema multiforme?

Immune complex hypersensitivity reaction to various causative agents

**What are the various causes of erythema multiforme?**

Half of all cases are idiopathic but other causes are:

Infections

Bacterial (*Streptococcus, Mycoplasma*)

Viral (herpes simplex, hepatitis A or B)
Fungal

Drugs: nonsteroidal anti-inflammatory drugs (NSAIDs), penicillin, sulfonamides, thiazide diuretics, barbiturates, phenytoin

Malignancy

Collagen vascular disease

**What is the pathopneumonic lesion?**

Erythematous **target lesions** with red center and dark outer ring in many different shapes (that is why it is called multiforme) (Fig 11-8)

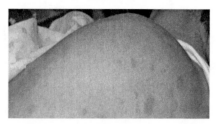

**Figure 11-8**    Target lesions. (Courtesy of Noah Craft, MD, PhD)

**Where are lesions mostly found?**

On the palms, soles, and extremities

**What forms can the lesions take?**

Many forms—vesicles, papules, bullae

**What is the treatment?**

Treat the underlying cause. Stop any drugs causing the reaction or treat any underlying infection.

**What is Stevens-Johnson syndrome?**

A severe form of erythema multiforme with systemic symptoms as well as **mucous membrane** involvement (oral mucosa and conjunctiva); <10% of body; potentially fatal (Fig 11-9)

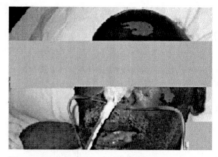

**Figure 11-9**    Stevens-Johnson syndrome. (Courtesy of Noah Craft, MD, PhD)

**What is the treatment?**

Remove/treat causative agent; systemic corticosteroid therapy; treat skin lesions as burns; immune globulin intravenous (IGIV) potentially helpful

**What can Stevens-Johnson syndrome progress to?**

Toxic epidermal necrolysis (TEN)

**How is TEN different from Stevens-Johnson?**

>30% of body surface area with full-thickness skin necrosis; higher risk of being fatal

**What happens to the target lesions in TEN?**

Lesions become confluent, tender, erythematous, and become bullae. There is eventual loss of the epidermis.

**What is "positive" sign for TEN?**

Nikolsky sign—Gentle manual traction leads to sloughing off of epidermis.

**What is the treatment?**

Remove/treat causative agent (acyclovir to prevent herpes recurrence); fluid and electrolyte replacement; systemic corticosteroids; IGIV may be helpful

**What is erythema nodosum?**

A painful inflammation of subcutaneous fat

**What is the etiology?**

Most cases are idiopathic.

Other causes:

**Drugs:** oral contraceptives, sulfonamides

**Infections:** *Streptococcus*, TB, leprosy, *Chlamydia*

**Autoimmune:** inflammatory bowel disease, Behçet, sarcoidosis, rheumatic fever, pregnancy

**In what patient population is it most commonly seen?**

Young women between the ages of 15 and 30

**What is seen on physical examination?**

**Erythematous nodules on lower legs that are extremely tender to touch**

(Note: Nodules are bilateral but not symmetric. Occasionally found on forearms or other areas with fat.) (Fig 11-10)

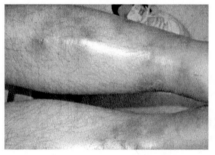

**Figure 11-10**   Erythema nodosum. (Courtesy of Noah Craft, MD, PhD)

**How is the diagnosis confirmed?**

CBC, CXR, throat culture, antistreptolysin-O

**What is the treatment?**

Treat the underlying cause as well as anti-inflammatories for pain and leg elevation.

**What is pityriasis rosea? And what is the sequence of eruption?**

A self-limiting maculopapular pruritic rash with central scale that begins as a **single herald patch** on the trunk, then followed by a generalized rash of pink scaly patches within 2 weeks of the initial eruption. Caused by HHV-7. (Fig 11-11)

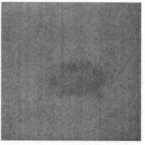

**Figure 11-11**  Herald patch in pityriasis rosea. (Courtesy of Noah Craft, MD, PhD)

**What is the pattern of distribution of the generalized rash?**

**Christmas tree pattern** on the back (Fig 11-12)

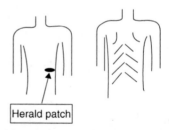

Herald patch

**Figure 11-12**  Herald patch and Christmas tree pattern.

**In what season is this most commonly seen?**

Spring

**In what patient population does it most commonly present?**

Children and young adults

**What is the treatment?**

Treatment is symptomatic only; it usually self-resolves in 6-8 weeks; however, sunlight helps.

Symptomatic treatment includes antihistamines, topical corticosteroids, and calamine lotion.

What is scabies?

An infection by the *Sarcoptes scabiei* mite which causes an extremely pruritic papular rash. Lesions are contagious.

What should you look for on physical examination if you suspect scabies?

Burrows in webs of finger, toes, and other intertriginous areas

How is it diagnosed?

Microscopic identification of the *S scabiei* mite in skin scraping

What is the treatment?

Permethrin 5% cream to entire body for 8 hours, then repeat 1 week later. Wash all linens. Antihistamines can help with pruritis.

How long can postscabies pruritis last after treatment?

6-8 weeks after treatment

Who should be treated?

Patient with scabies and all close contacts

# CLINICAL VIGNETTES

An obese 37-year-old diabetic, hyperlipidemic male presents to your clinic for a follow-up. His HgA1c is 8. His LDL is 100 and HDL is 40. He complains of a dark "rash" that has slowly appeared in the posterior fold of his neck. It is nonpruritic, and not painful. On examination there is an area of hyperpigmented skin that has a "velvety" texture to it. What is the most likely diagnosis?

Acanthosis nigricans

In the month of March, a healthy 23-year-old female presents to your office complaining of a very pruritic rash. She states that the rash started as a single larger lesion; then about 5 days later she broke out in a rash on her entire back that is extremely pruritic. She has not started any new medications or used any new products either. This has never happened to her in the past. On examination you find a single larger scaly lesion on her upper back and a generalized rash consisting of pink scaly patches. Her vitals are within normal limits. What is the most likely diagnosis?

Pityriasis rosea

A 17-year-old male presents complaining of some lesions on his back. He states that they do not cause him any discomfort. There is no itching or pain. On examination you find small, hypopigmented patches on his upper back. With scratching there is fine overlying scale. A KOH preparation shows pseudohyphae and yeast. What is the organism causing his rash?

*Malassezia furfur* is the organism in tinea versicolor.

An 87-year-old female who lives in a convalescent home is brought in for evaluation of a rash. The rash is extremely pruritic, especially in the evening. The caretaker mentions that her roommate has similar symptoms. The patient has a generalized rash with a lot of excoriation marks on her body. When you look in the webs of her fingers you find superficial burrows. What is the most likely diagnosis?

Scabies

A fair-skinned 57-year-old construction worker presents for a skin check. On the helix of his ear you find red, scaly rough patches. They are then treated with liquid nitrogen. What are these lesions precursors of?

SCC

# CHAPTER 12

# Clinical Vignettes Review

A 45-year-old female who recently had surgery for a thyroid cancer develops perioral paresthesias, confusion, and muscle weakness. An EKG was performed and it demonstrated a prolonged QT interval. What is the most likely reason for this woman's symptoms?

Hypocalcemia

A 30-year-old African-American female presents to your office complaining of a photosensitive skin rash over her nose and cheeks as well as fever and polyarthritis. She reports no pain. You listen to her heart and hear a murmur. Based on the previous findings, what do you think is the most likely cause of the murmur?

Libman-Sacks endocarditis (Mnemonic: SLE causes LSE)

A 60-year-old alcoholic female presents with severe back pain with nausea and vomiting. Abdominal x-ray shows a sentinel loop. What is the most likely diagnosis?

Pancreatitis

A patient diagnosed with leukemia has Auer rods on blood smear. What type of leukemia does he have?

Acute myelogenous leukemia (AML)

A young boy presents to the dentist and is found to have excessive bleeding. Laboratory tests are performed and he is found to have a prolonged bleeding time with normal prothrombin time (PT)/partial prothrombin time (PTT). What is the diagnosis of choice?

von Willebrand disease

A 58-year-old female presents with acute renal failure of unknown etiology. Urinalysis shows Bence Jones proteinuria and she is found to have a monoclonal gammopathy. What is the diagnosis?

Multiple myeloma

A 70-year-old male in the intensive care unit (ICU) on total parenteral nutrition (TPN) for 10 days develops jaundice. Liver function test demonstrates a total bilirubin of 12. What is the most likely cause of his hyperbilirubinemia?

Cholestasis caused by parenteral nutrition

A 60-year-old female is found to be hypotensive on pressors with minimal improvement. Her chest x-ray (CXR) demonstrates an enlarged heart that resembles a water bottle. What would be the test you would order to make the diagnosis?

Echocardiogram. This patient most likely has a pericardial effusion.

A 50-year-old male who had a myocardial infarction (MI) approximately 3 weeks prior presents with fever and elevated erythrocyte sedimentation rate (ESR). What is the most likely diagnosis?

Dressler syndrome

You are called by the nurse about a hospitalized patient with a blood pressure of 100/60. You go to evaluate the patient and on examination she has distant heart sounds and jugular venous distention (JVD). You order an EKG and you notice that the height of the QRS complex varies from beat to beat. What is your diagnosis?

Cardiac tamponade

An otherwise healthy medical student gets his annual purified protein derivative (PPD) (tuberculin) as required by medical school; 48 hours later he goes to have it read and it measures 10 mm. What would you tell this student about the results?

He has a positive PPD and needs to be treated with 6-9 months of isoniazid (INH).

A 30-year-old female presents with fatigue for several months. She has also had multiple urinary tract infections (UTIs) over the past year. You order a complete blood count (CBC) with a peripheral smear. The smear shows Auer rods and 52% myeloblasts. What is the diagnosis?

Acute myelocytic leukemia

A 60-year-old male presents to your office for a physical examination. He has no past medical history, does not drink or smoke, and currently takes no medications. His physical examination is benign except that he appears somewhat pale. His CBC shows a hemoglobin of 11 and the mean corpuscular volume (MCV) is 70. He has a low ferritin, low serum iron, and elevated total iron-binding capacity (TIBC). What is your next step?

Screen for colon cancer—Iron deficiency anemia is colon cancer until proven otherwise.

Your 16-year-old patient comes to your office because his friends told him that he looks "yellow." He has no past medical history and is not taking any medications. He denies any recent antibiotic use. He does mention that he has felt fatigued over the past 2 days. He also says that he tried Indian food for the first time a few days ago. He had a really tasty bean dish. You order a CBC and his hemoglobin is 8. What is the diagnosis?

Glucose-6-phosphate dehydrogenase (G6PD) deficiency

An HIV patient with a CD4 count of 198 comes to see you for follow-up on his HIV. What new antibiotic would you initiate?

Bactrim as prophylaxis against *Pneumocystis carinii* pneumonia (PCP)

A 55-year-old alcoholic male is brought in to the emergency room (ER) for altered mental status. He is found to have a pulse oxygen of 85%. A stat CXR is done and the patient is found to have a large right upper lobe consolidation. He is reported to have a "currant jelly" sputum. What is the most likely organism?

*Klebsiella* secondary to an aspiration pneumonia

A 25-year-old female presents to your office complaining of diarrhea, weight loss, and heart palpitations. What initial test would you order?

Thyroid-stimulating hormone (TSH) and T4

(Think: hyperthyroidism)

A 70-year-old male presents with renal failure. During your history and physical on your review of systems you discover that he has been having bone pain and weight loss over the past several months. On your initial laboratory assessment you find that your patient is hypercalcemic, has rouleaux formation, and has Bence Jones proteins in his urine. A serum protein electrophoresis demonstrates an "M" spike. You order an x-ray and find he has "punched out lesions." What is the most likely diagnosis?

Multiple myeloma

A patient presents to the ER with symptoms of nausea, vomiting, and fatigue. He tells you that over the past few months he has had a significant amount of weight loss. His sister, who has come to the hospital with him, says that she has noticed that recently his skin has become very tanned as well. You question the patient about recent sun exposure and he tells you that he has had very little since he is an accountant and is indoors most of the day. His laboratory tests reveal that he is hyponatremic and hyperkalemic. What diagnostic test would you order for this patient?

Plasma adrenocorticotropic hormone (ACTH) level to evaluate for Addison disease

A patient with a history of IV drug abuse presents to the hospital with high fever and chills. On physical examination you hear a new murmur. Blood cultures are drawn and are positive × 2 with *Streptococcus viridans*. What is the most likely diagnosis?

Endocarditis. The tricuspid valve is most likely involved.

Unfortunately, your patient has been diagnosed with lung cancer. He has been feeling very weak and fatigued for the past few days and develops an altered level of consciousness. A CT scan was done and fortunately there were no metastases to the brain. Electrolytes show that he has a sodium of 125. His glucose is within normal limits. What test would you order next to confirm your suspected diagnosis?

Urine electrolytes to confirm the most likely diagnosis of SIADH (syndrome of inappropriate antidiuretic hormone)

A nursing home patient who is alert and oriented presents with severe hyponatremia. Your colleague treats the patient with hypertonic saline and is able to correct his sodium within 7 hours. Subsequently, the patient becomes unresponsive and unarousable. Your colleague does not know what happened. What would you tell her was the cause of her patient's rapid alteration in mental status?

The patient has central pontine myelinolysis. Hyponatremia should never be corrected too quickly for this reason.

A patient in renal failure complains of chest pain. Her potassium is 6.5. A stat EKG shows peaked T waves. What would be the initial treatment that should be given?

Calcium gluconate to protect the heart

Your next patient in clinic is a 75-year-old white male visiting for a routine physical. He mentions that he has noticed a lesion on the ridge of his ear. You take a look at it and find it is pearly in appearance and has some telangiectasias. What is the most likely diagnosis?

Basal cell carcinoma

A sexually active 18-year-old male presents with a hot, swollen, severely painful right knee for the past 2 days. He denies any history of trauma to the joint that he can recall. What is the next step in diagnosis?

Arthrocentesis. Most likely organism is *Neisseria gonorrhoeae*.

A 77-year-old female complains of severe joint pain over the past several years. On her hands you notice some nodules on her proximal interphalangeal joints (PIP). What are these nodules called?

Bouchard nodes

A 45-year-old woman presents to the ER complaining of dyspnea and chest pain. She just came back from a cross-country road trip. She also tells you that she had one episode of hemoptysis. The nurse takes her vitals. They are: Tmax: 37.8°C; BP: 130/90; pulse: 110; respiratory rate: 28; and oxygen saturation of 88%. You examine the patient and find that her left calf is swollen and tender. What is the most likely diagnosis for this patient's shortness of breath?

Pulmonary embolism from a deep venous thrombosis (DVT) in her left lower extremity

A 20-year-old patient presents with altered level of consciousness. His parents report that he has been very thirsty recently. A serum glucose is 849. What test could you order to differentiate between type 1 and type 2 diabetes?

C-peptide. It would be missing in type 1 diabetics.

A 45-year-old obese female presents with a 2-day history of nausea, vomiting, and abdominal pain. On examination the patient has right upper quadrant pain. You suspect cholecystitis so you order a right upper quadrant ultrasound. The test is equivocal. What is your next step in management?

This patient needs a hydroxy iminodiacetic acid (HIDA) scan.

A 70-year-old male with a 35-pack-year history of smoking presents with dyspnea on exertion. The patient has a chronic dry cough and his voice sounds very hoarse. Physical examination demonstrates decreased breath sounds, a hyper-resonant chest, and distant heart sounds. A CXR reveals flattened diaphragms. What is the diagnosis?

Chronic obstructive pulmonary disease (COPD)

A 25-year-old male presents with acute right knee pain. The patient denies any history of trauma but does report fever and chills. He also tells you that over the last week he has had pain in multiple joints as well. He admits to you that he is sexually active with multiple partners and does not like to use any protection. On physical examination, the knee is swollen, erythematous, and painful. He has a rash on his palms. You tap the joint and the fluid demonstrates gram-negative diplococci. What is the diagnosis?

Gonococcal arthritis

An 84-year-old male with a past medical history significant for hypertension, hyperlipidemia, and diabetes presents with left-sided paralysis. He is admitted to the hospital for further workup. In the next 15 hours, his symptoms resolve. What is the most likely diagnosis?

Transient ischemie attack (TIA)

A 19-year-old male presents to your clinic complaining of a "rash" on his knees and elbows. He says that he has used moisturizer on it with no improvement. On physical examination, you find silvery white scaly patches on his elbows and knees. You also notice that he has pitting of some of his fingernails. What is the most likely diagnosis?

Psoriasis

A young male presents with a 3-month history of night sweats, fatigue, and 15-lb weight loss. He has noticed that he has a single, nontender cervical lymph node that does not seem to be resolving. He did mention that his symptoms seem worse with alcohol consumption. A CBC demonstrates leukocytosis. A lymph node biopsy demonstrates binucleated giant cells (Reed-Sternberg cells). What is the diagnosis?

Hodgkin lymphoma

A patient presents with altered mental status with petechiae on the lower extremities. The patient has a temperature of 38.3°C, blood pressure of 110/80. The following are the patient's labs: CBC: WBC 10, hemoglobin 10, hematocrit 26, and platelets 50. Electrolytes demonstrates hyperkalemia and blood urea nitrogen/creatine (BUN/CR) of 40/2.5. The patient has an elevated lactate dehydrogenase (LDH) and unconjugated bilirubin. What is the diagnosis?

Thrombotic thrombocytopenic purpura (TTP)

An 18-year-old athlete presents with an erythematous, pruritic skin eruption in the intertriginous region. A potassium hydroxide (KOH) scraping demonstrates hyphae. What is the diagnosis?

Tinea cruris

An HIV patient presents with purple-colored macules and nodules on his skin. It is caused by human herpesvirus 8 (HHV 8). What is the diagnosis?

Kaposi sarcoma